Alzheimer's at your fingertips

THE COMPREHENSIVE DEMENTIA REFERENCE BOOK FOR THE YEAR 2000

Harry Cayton, BA, BPhil, Dip Anth
Executive Director of the Alzheimer's Disease Society

Dr. Nori Graham, BM BCh, FRCPsych, D Univ
Consultant in Old Age Psychiatry, Royal Free Hospital, London and Chairman of Alzheimer's Disease International

Dr. James Warner, BSc, MB BS, MRCP, MRCPsych
Lecturer in Psychiatry, Royal Free Hospital School of Medicine, London

D0273821

CLASS PUBLISHING • LONDON

Harry Cayton, Nori Graham and James Warner assert their rights as set out in Sections 77 and 78 of the Copyright, Designs and Patents Act 1988 to be identified as the authors of this work wherever it is published commercially and whenever any adaptation of this work is published or produced including any sound recordings or films based upon this work.

Printing history
First published 1997
Reprinted 1998
Reprinted with revisions 1998

The authors and publishers welcome feedback from the users of this book. Please contact the publishers.

Class Publishing, Barb House, Barb Mews, London W6 7PA, UK
Telephone: 0171 371 2119
Fax: 0171 371 2878 [International +44171]
email: post@class.co.uk
http: www.class.co.uk

A CIP catalogue record for this book is available from the British Library

ISBN 1 872362 71 0

Designed by Wendy Bann

Edited and typeset by Ruth Midgley

Cartoons by Linda Moore

Illustration by David Woodroffe

Production by Landmark Production Consultants Ltd, Princes Risborough

Printed and bound in Finland by WSOY

Contents

Foreword

by Dr. JONATHAN MILLER, CBE
President of the Alzheimer's Disease Society

There can be few situations more distressing than watching the gradual mental disintegration of a parent, partner or friend as they drift away into the grip of Alzheimer's disease. Alzheimer's disease and the other dementias may destroy the sense of past and of present in the person who has the disease but they can also shatter the lives of those who care for them.

The burden for carers is great: physical, mental and emotional. But all burdens can be shared. The experience of other carers, knowledge of dementias and knowing where to get help all make the caring task easier.

That is where this book makes an invaluable contribution to understanding all forms of dementia. It is down to earth, sensible and realistic. It deals with very many of the questions you may want to ask and gives straightforward, practical answers. The format of *Alzheimer's at your fingertips* means that you can dip into it as and when you want to and quickly find the answer to the problem you have at that time.

Between them the authors of this book have great experience of looking after people with dementia and helping their carers. In compiling the questions to be answered they have drawn on the ideas and interests of carers themselves. As President of the Alzheimer's Disease Society I know how important bringing together professionals and family members to share knowledge and experience can be. This book will be essential for all those involved in caring for people with dementia and advising their families.

Jonathan Miller

Acknowledgements

In writing this book we have drawn on our own experience and reading and are grateful to all our colleagues for their advice. In particular the Alzheimer's Disease Society's publications have been an invaluable source of clear and accurate information. A number of colleagues have read and commented on the text as we have gone along. Responsibility for the content of the book is however ours and ours alone.

We extend special thanks to the following people:

Dr. Martin Blanchard, BSc, MB BS, MD, MRCPsych, Senior Lecturer in Old Age Psychiatry, Honorary Consultant, Royal Free Hospital School of Medicine

Janice Brown, Publications Officer, Alzheimer's Disease Society

Ruth Finch and members of the Hammersmith branch of the Alzheimer's Disease Society

Marjorie King for secretarial support

Helen Krizka and members of the Camden support group of the Alzheimer's Disease Society for providing many of the questions

Steve Milton, Information Officer, Alzheimer's Disease Society

Introduction

If you are a carer or if you know someone with dementia this book is for you. The confusion which is the main feature of dementia does not only affect the person with the condition. Carers, family members and friends are also bewildered and confused by the behaviour of the person they know. Often when the diagnosis is first made you do not think of all the questions that you want to ask or you may feel you are not ready to ask them. But as time passes you will probably want to know as much as possible about dementia and how to care for someone who has it. Knowledge is the best way of lifting the cloud of confusion and taking charge of the situation for yourself.

Although this book is written mainly for family carers it will also be useful for care-workers in the community and in residential and nursing homes. Many of the questions answered, particularly about communication, behaviour and treatments, are the same whoever you are or wherever you are working. Some people who have been given a diagnosis of dementia may also find parts of the book useful, perhaps particularly those on dementia itself and on legal and financial arrangements. As earlier diagnosis is achieved, more people with dementia will want and will be able to plan their own treatment and care in agreement with their families.

This book is called *Alzheimer's at your fingertips* but it is about all the dementias not just Alzheimer's disease. Alzheimer's disease is the commonest type of dementia and the name has become widely used by the public as a general term for what was formerly known, wrongly, as senile dementia. In this book the term Alzheimer's disease is used only to refer to that particular form of dementia. Most of the questions and answers, however, will be relevant whatever form of dementia you are concerned with.

The book answers 266 questions. All the questions are real questions asked by carers, by friends and family members and by people with dementia themselves. We have tried to answer them as clearly and as accurately as we can. Research into Alzheimer's disease is moving fast, new drug treatments are becoming available and, of course, the law on social security is subject to change, so you may need to check on the details if you are using this book some time after it was published.

You will probably not want to read this book from cover to cover. Some chapters will be relevant to you at different stages of the condition. The usefulness of some parts will depend on the type of dementia which concerns you, or on your financial circumstances, or on your relationship to the person you care for. This is a book to be referred to as and when you need to. We hope it will be easy to dip into. Each question and answer is self-contained and there are cross references to other questions and answers whenever that seems helpful.

Chapters 1 and 2 in *Alzheimer's at your fingertips* answer questions about the different types and causes of dementia. Chapters 3 to 8 aim to help you with the practical issues of looking after someone with dementia. In chapter 9 we explain where you can get help and in 11 the financial and legal arrangements which can be made to aid you. Chapter 10 looks at care in residential and nursing homes. Chapter 12 describes different types of treatment while the final chapter looks to current and future research.

No one book on dementia is ever going to be enough. We have added a reading list of other publications which we hope will be helpful to you. There is also an appendix including the names and addresses of some useful organisations.

It isn't easy caring for someone with dementia but, as we hope this book shows, many difficulties can be overcome. Sharing your problems and feelings with others is perhaps the most important thing you can do. Organisations like the Alzheimer's Disease Society, Alzheimer Scotland and the Alzheimer's Society of Ireland are there with information, practical help and emotional support.

Future editions of *Alzheimer's at your fingertips* can only be improved if you let us know if you would like to add to any of our answers or if you think we could offer other useful advice. We would also like to know if there are important questions that we have not included. Please write to the authors c/o Class Publishing, Barb House, Barb Mews, London W6 7PA, UK.

1
What is Alzheimer's disease?

Introduction

Alzheimer's disease is the most common type of dementia. This chapter tells you about Alzheimer's disease, what we know about its causes, how it damages the brain, and its affect on people who have it. Although there are many similarities between different types of dementia, it helps to distinguish between them and to understand the differences. The more we know about Alzheimer's disease, the better care we can give.

Defining Alzheimer's disease

Where did Alzheimer's disease get its name?

Alzheimer's disease is named after Dr Alois Alzheimer, a German neurologist (1864-1915), who in 1906 observed changes in the brain tissue of a woman who had died of what was thought to be an unusual mental illness. These abnormal brain tissue changes are now known to be the characteristic features of Alzheimer's disease.

The term dementia sometimes seems to be used instead of Alzheimer's disease. Are they two names for the same thing?

Dementia is a term used to describe various disorders of the brain that all result in progressive and severe loss of memory. Alzheimer's disease is the most common type of dementia, accounting on its own for approximately 50% of all cases (and occurring with another cause in a further 20% of cases). Alzheimer's disease also causes certain specific changes to the brain tissue (see the next answer).

People with Alzheimer's disease (and other dementias), gradually lose their sense of time and place. A major symptom is that they forget things that they have just said or done, although their memory for past events may for a time remain clear. As the disease progresses, people become unaware of their condition although they may still experience distress. They find it increasingly difficult and then impossible to perform even the simplest everyday tasks, including washing, eating and dressing, without supervision. They may become uncommunicative and incontinent, sometimes with severe behavioural problems. Most eventually need 24-hour care. The disease may go on for many years – typically between five and 10 years – and tends not to be the eventual cause of death. More commonly, a person has Alzheimer's disease for many years before dying from something else, such as an infection or stroke.

Is it true that the only certain way of knowing if someone has had Alzheimer's disease is to carry out a post mortem examination of the brain?

In most cases, an absolutely certain diagnosis of Alzheimer's disease usually depends on finding characteristic changes in the brain tissue. These changes can only be found during the course of a post mortem examination. Spread throughout the brains of people who have died of Alzheimer's disease are deposits, or plaques, made up of an abnormal protein called beta amyloid. A further abnormality is the occurrence of tangles of twisted protein molecules within the nerve cells of the brain. Other features, also found in other dementias, are shrinkage of the brain and widespread death of cells.

In rare cases, where a person has a gene that is known to cause an inherited form of Alzheimer's disease (see p. 4), a test for that gene can confirm the diagnosis.

However, in practice, the diagnosis of Alzheimer's disease is usually made on the basis of identifying that a person is suffering from some form of dementia, and then ruling out various conditions other than Alzheimer's disease that might be the cause. (See Chapter 3 for more about diagnosis.)

What is the difference between senile dementia and Alzheimer's disease?

The term senile dementia was formerly used when people 'lost their memory' at an older age. This loss of memory was thought to be part of the normal ageing process. However, it is now appreciated that most people do not develop dementia even at a great age. Most of what used to be called senile dementia was in fact Alzheimer's disease.

Alzheimer's disease is the same disease at whatever age it occurs. In the past, however, a distinction used to be made on the basis of age. Older people were described as having senile dementia, while younger ones were said to have pre-senile dementia. This distinction is now widely considered unhelpful and misleading and these terms are strongly discouraged.

Who will get Alzheimer's disease?

A lot of people now seem to be developing Alzheimer's disease. How common is it? And is it on the increase?

Alzheimer's disease is uncommon in younger people but becomes more common with age. It can affect people as young as 30, but this is very rare. Up to the age of 65, Alzheimer's disease develops in only about one person in 1,000. In older people, the disease becomes more common, affecting around three people in 100 over the age of 65. Over the age of 80, this figure rises to between 10 and 15 per 100.

The numbers of people who currently have Alzheimer's disease in the UK is approaching 400,000 (while a further 300,000 have other forms of dementia). These numbers are increasing. This increase is due partly to earlier diagnosis but mainly to the fact that more people are now living longer and reaching an age at which the risk of developing Alzheimer's disease is increased.

Is Alzheimer's disease more common in some groups of people than others?

As far as is known, Alzheimer's disease occurs equally across all groups in society. It is not known to be linked with gender, social class, ethnic group or geographic location. Alzheimer's disease is more common in older age groups and in people with Down's syndrome (see p. 7).

Does Alzheimer's disease run in families?

Alzheimer's disease does sometimes run in families, but this is uncommon. Some rare cases of the disease, which tend to occur in younger people than usual, are known to be passed on in the genes from one generation to the next (see the next answer and p. 6). In these cases, the probability that close family members (brothers, sisters and children) will develop Alzheimer's disease is one in two.

Most cases of Alzheimer's disease are not of the type that is passed on genetically. If a family member suffers from the non-genetic form of the disease, the risk to close relatives is around three times higher than the risk for a person of a similar age who has no family history of the disease. It is thought that in these cases a person's genes may contribute to the development of the disease but do not cause it directly.

How would I know if my family has the inherited form of Alzheimer's disease? And how likely would this make me to get the disease?

The form of Alzheimer's disease that is definitely known to be passed on from one generation to the next in the genes is extremely rare. It is very unlikely that your family has it unless close relatives have developed the disease below the age of 60. This form of Alzheimer's disease develops at a younger age than usual, typically between the ages of 35 and 60, and tends to develop at a similar age within the family.

If your family does have this inherited form of Alzheimer's disease, you are only at risk if your mother or father developed it. If one of them did develop it, you have a one in two chance of developing the disease. In these circumstances, a genetic test (see p. 39) could be requested to confirm whether or not you do in fact have the gene for this disease.

Causes of Alzheimer's disease

How much is known about the possible causes of Alzheimer's disease?

This is an important area of current research, but at the present time a great deal still remains to be discovered about why people develop Alzheimer's disease.

We know that Alzheimer's disease becomes more common with increasing age, but we don't know what factors trigger the characteristic changes that occur in the brain tissue of people who have this disease. We know that these brain changes are associated with ageing, but also that they are not part of the normal ageing process. In some cases, the changes occur at a relatively early age.

Genes are thought to play a part in the development of most cases of Alzheimer's disease. In rare cases, abnormal genes actually cause the disease. Much more commonly, genes are believed only to contribute to a person's susceptibility to the disease. It seems that, at least in some cases, factors in the environment may be necessary to trigger the illness.

Alzheimer's disease is certainly not infectious. Nor is it caused by over-use or under-use of the brain. Even though the disease is sometimes first noticed after a period of stress or worry, it is not thought that these emotions can actually cause the disease to develop. Nor is it believed that the trauma of an operation can trigger the disease. Claims are sometimes made that dietary or hormone deficiencies may contribute to the development of Alzheimer's disease, but most doctors do not accept these claims. Similarly, claims that aluminium in the diet may be a cause (see p. 7) are not widely accepted.

How do genes cause Alzheimer's disease?

Research suggests that the genes associated with the development of Alzheimer's disease might have a detrimental effect on chemicals known as neurotransmitters, which allow messages to be communicated between nerve cells. One type of neurotransmitter, called acetylcholine, is known to be deficient in Alzheimer's disease.

Another way in which abnormal genes might exert their effect is through their influence on nerve growth factor. It is thought that genes might interfere with the way that this factor normally enhances the growth of functioning nerve cells to compensate for the death of other cells.

Recently, research has focussed on a gene which makes a protein called apolipoprotein E (ApoE). There are three types of ApoE – E2, E3, E4. Each person inherits an ApoE gene from each parent. It seems that people who inherit an ApoE-E4 gene have a higher risk of developing Alzheimer's disease.

Abnormalities on three other genes – PS1 (presenilin amyloid precursor protein, type 1), PS2 and APP (amyloid precursor protein) – have also been identified as causes of the rare inherited form of the disease, but the mechanism is not clear.

Why do people with Down's syndrome develop Alzheimer's disease?

People with Down's syndrome usually have an extra chromosome 21. One gene on chromosome 21 codes for amyloid precursor protein (APP). Abnormal deposition of amyloid in the brain occurs in Alzheimer's disease. It seems the extra gene results in an excess of amyloid. Consequently, almost all people with Down's syndrome over age forty develop the characteristic brain tissue changes of Alzheimer's disease.

Does aluminium cause Alzheimer's disease? Is it safe to use aluminium saucepans?

This is a controversial issue. A number of research findings have suggested a possible link between aluminium and Alzheimer's disease. These findings include: the presence of aluminium deposits in tangles and plaques (see p. 3) in the brains of people with Alzheimer's disease; and increased rates of dementia in people with kidney failure whose bodies have raised levels of aluminium. However, a large study of the brains of people who had died from Alzheimer's disease did not find higher than normal levels of aluminium.

Some studies have suggested that people living in areas with high concentrations of aluminium in the water supply may be more likely to develop Alzheimer's disease. However, this evidence is inconclusive. Exposure to aluminium from other sources, such as from drinking tea, using antiperspirants and taking antacids has not been shown to be linked to the development of Alzheimer's disease.

Since there is only weak or circumstantial evidence for linking aluminium with the development of Alzheimer's disease, there would seem to be little justification for not using aluminium cooking utensils.

Might mercury in dental fillings cause Alzheimer's?

This is not thought to be likely, but more research is awaited. Mercury has been shown to be toxic to the central nervous system, but this does not prove any link with Alzheimer's disease. Nor is a link proved by unconfirmed research that suggests the brains of people with Alzheimer's disease might contain more mercury than normal.

Is it possible to take precautions against developing Alzheimer's disease?

Not enough is known yet about the causes of Alzheimer's disease (see p. 5) for any precautions to be recommended.

Symptoms and signs

How do the early symptoms of Alzheimer's disease differ from ordinary forgetfulness?

Many older people find that their memories are not as good as they used to be. For example, they have difficulty remembering people's names, things they were going to buy, or something they were going to do. This does not mean that they are getting Alzheimer's disease. A person who is ordinarily forgetful can still remember details associated with the thing they have forgotten. For example, they may briefly forget their next door neighbour's name but they still know that the person they are talking to is their neighbour. People with Alzheimer's disease forget not only details but the entire context. They may also have other problems, such as changes in behaviour and loss of ability to do everyday tasks.

What are the tell-tale signs of the onset of Alzheimer's disease? What should I be looking out for?

One of the changes that often appears in the early stages of Alzheimer's disease is that the person seems different from their usual self, but in ways that are hard to pinpoint. The person seems less capable, less involved and less adaptable. You may notice that they lose interest in hobbies and pastimes. They may show loss of concentration, may be unable to make decisions and seem to avoid taking responsibility. They may also show some odd behaviours, such as getting ready to go to work many years after they have retired. The person may be showing odd mood changes, such as irritability and suspicion, which may be due to becoming aware that something is wrong but not knowing quite what the problem is. All these changes are quite difficult to pick up early on. They are more often identified when looking back and trying to work out what the first signs of the disease were.

Does Alzheimer's disease differ from one person to another?

Alzheimer's disease does affect people differently. Although the disease tends to follow a broadly similar pattern – a progressive decline in mental capabilities over a number of years – its impact is affected by what a person was like in the first place. Personality, physical condition and social situation can all be important. Some people become increasingly disagreeable and difficult to live with, whereas others become more sweet-natured and amenable. Some people with Alzheimer's disease have few other health problems, whereas others have disabilities – such as arthritis or deafness – that can make their care more difficult. Some people have a comparatively comfortable social situation, whereas others are faced with family or financial problems.

How does Alzheimer's disease usually progress? Does it always follow the same course?

No two people with Alzheimer's disease will follow exactly the same course. The disease will progress more quickly in some people than others, and no one will experience all of the symptoms and signs listed here. It is also important to point out that the disease typically progresses gradually and does not fit neatly into the three stages outlined here. Even so, it can be helpful to look at the typical symptoms and signs of Alzheimer's disease in the context of three stages of development – early, middle and late. These stages will serve as a rough guide to the most likely progression of the disease and may help carers to be aware of potential problems and to make plans for future care needs.

Early symptoms
The early stage of Alzheimer's disease is often overlooked, being incorrectly labelled by professionals, relatives and friends as 'old age' or a normal part of the process of ageing. Because the onset of the disease is gradual, it is difficult to identify exactly when it begins. The person may:
- show difficulties with language;
- experience significant memory loss – having particular problems with short-term memory;
- be disorientated in time;
- become lost in familiar places;
- display difficulty in making decisions;
- lack initiative and motivation;
- show signs of depression and aggression;
- show a loss of interest in hobbies and activities.

Middle symptoms
As the disease progresses, problems become more evident and restricting. The person with Alzheimer's disease has difficulty with day-to-day living, and:
- may become very forgetful – especially of recent events and people's names;

- can no longer manage to live alone without problems;
- is unable to cook, clean or shop;
- may become extremely dependent;
- needs assistance with personal hygiene, including visiting the toilet, bathing and washing;
- needs help with dressing;
- has increased difficulty with speech;
- wanders and sometimes gets lost;
- shows various behavioural abnormalities, such as unprovoked aggression or constantly following the carer around the house;
- may experience hallucinations.

Late symptoms
This stage is one of total dependence and inactivity. Memory disturbances are very serious and the physical side of the disease becomes more obvious. The person may:
- have difficulty eating;
- not recognise relatives, friends and familiar objects;
- have difficulty understanding and interpreting events;
- be unable to find his or her way around in the home;
- have difficulty walking;
- suffer bladder and bowel incontinence;
- display inappropriate behaviour in public;
- be confined to a wheelchair or bed.

Why is it that my wife, who has dementia, is able to remember things from years ago but can't remember what happened half an hour ago?

There are several linked processes involved in memory. First, an experience is perceived. It is then placed in a short-term memory store and retained for a brief time. If the experience recurs or is likely to be important, it goes into a long-term memory store. Finally, for a memory to be recaptured it must be recalled from a memory store.

People with dementia gradually lose the ability to enter new information into their memory. They also have difficulty in recalling previously stored memories. Memory for recent events is affected first. People with dementia tend to be better at recalling memories from long ago.

My wife no longer recognises me. Why is this?

This is a very painful experience that commonly occurs in the late stage of Alzheimer's disease. The likely explanation is that although your wife may be able to see your face, she is unable to link this to her memories of you and therefore does not recognise you.

Outlook

My doctor recently told me that my wife has Alzheimer's disease. Is it bound to get worse?

You will need to be prepared for a gradual worsening of your wife's condition over the years. Although there may be no apparent change between one month and the next, changes will be apparent between one year and the next. In general, most people with Alzheimer's disease become very forgetful and quite disabled within five years or so of the diagnosis.

One way of helping your wife to live as well as possible as the disease progresses is to ensure that she receives prompt treatment for any other medical problems, such as depression (see p. 163) or an infection. New drugs (p. 156) may temporarily slow the progress of the disease for some people.

It is useful for relatives and carers to know about the likely progression of the disease so that they are aware of what is going to happen and can help to prepare themselves and make plans for the future. You will need to consider the possibility of day care (p. 116), respite care (p. 117) and eventually residential care (see Chapter 10). Your doctor, community psychiatric nurse (p. 115) or a member of a local carers' self-help group (such as a local Alzheimer's Disease Society group) will be able to give you further advice.

2

Other dementias

Introduction

The term dementia covers a number of different diseases and disorders, with a range of different causes. The most common type of dementia is Alzheimer's disease (covered in Chapter 1). This chapter provides information on other dementias, including vascular dementia (see p. 19), which is the second commonest type, as well as a wide of range of less common types.

Defining dementia

What is dementia?

Dementia is a term used to describe a group of different brain disorders that resemble each other in causing a progressive and severe loss of memory.

People with dementia have particular problems with their short-term memory. They consistently forget things that they have just said or done, even though they can often recall clearly events that happened many years ago. Their sense of time and place is typically lost. They may develop problems with finding words and it becomes increasingly difficult for them to learn new information and to do new things. As time goes on, people with dementia need help to perform even the most basic tasks of everyday living, including washing, dressing and eating. Eventually, people with dementia may become uncommunicative and incontinent. Sometimes there are severe behavioural problems. Most people with dementia eventually require 24-hour care. Dementias often go on for many years – five, 10 or even 20 – and are not usually the actual cause of death.

My family tell me that my grandmother became 'senile' in her last years. Does this mean she had senile dementia or could she have had Alzheimer's disease?

People quite often use the term 'senile' to describe old people who have become weak and confused in their thoughts. Strictly speaking, the word senile just means old, but people have often used it in common speech to mean senile dementia (a term that is itself falling out of use).

If your grandmother's 'senility' lasted for months or years before she died it is likely that she did have some form of dementia, probably Alzheimer's disease. However, if your grandmother's mental problems developed only in the last few weeks or months of her life it is more likely that she did not have a dementia but that her brain function was being affected by a disease elsewhere in the body, such as the liver, kidneys or heart.

At what age would someone be described as having pre-senile dementia rather than senile dementia?

Although these terms do sometimes still appear in textbooks, they are falling out of use and are being widely discouraged. In the past, the distinction tended to be made around age sixty. Senile dementia is just another term for dementia appearing in older people. Most of what used to be called pre-senile and senile dementia is in fact Alzheimer's disease.

I have been told that my next door neighbour has some sort of dementia but that she does not have Alzheimer's disease. What other dementias are there?

Dementia is a term used by doctors to describe a number of different diseases. All of these diseases affect the brain and cause a progressive loss of memory that eventually makes it impossible for the sufferer to perform even the simplest everyday tasks without help.

Alzheimer's disease (see Chapter 1) is the commonest type of dementia, accounting on its own for about half of all cases. There are, however, quite a number other types of dementia and it seems that your neighbour has been diagnosed with one of these. Among these other types of dementia, all but vascular dementia, which is the second commonest type of dementia, are rare.

Types of dementia other than Alzheimer's disease include:
- Vascular dementia (see p. 19), which results from brain damage due to tiny strokes;
- Pick's disease (see p. 20), in which there are striking changes in behaviour before the memory problems appear;
- Huntington's disease (see p. 21), also sometimes called Huntington's chorea, which is characterised by jerky movements in addition to dementia;
- AIDS-related dementia (see p. 22);

- Dementia that sometimes occurs together with Parkinson's disease (see p. 23);
- Lewy body disease (see p. 23), which some people regard as a variant of Alzheimer's disease or Parkinson's disease;
- Creutzfeld Jakob disease or CJD (see p. 24);
- Dementia due to a brain tumour (see p. 25);
- Normal pressure hydrocephalus, due to a build up of fluid in the brain (see p. 25);
- Dementia due to an excessive intake of alcohol over an extended period of time (see p. 25);
- Dementias due to various treatable causes, including vitamin deficiency (see p. 26), hormone deficiency (see 26), and syphilis.

Who will get dementia?

How common is dementia, and is it more common in some groups of people than others?

The chances of developing some form of dementia increase with age, but dementia does occur very rarely in people under the age of 60. Over the age of 65, dementia affects approximately six people in 100. For people over 80, the number affected rises to 20 in 100.

In general, dementia seems to affect all groups in society equally. It is not known to be linked with gender, social class, ethnic group or geographic location.

Causes of dementia

What are the causes of dementia?

Different types of dementia have different possible causes. In many cases, the causes are not fully understood. For example, dementia in general is much more common in older people, but the ageing process as such is not considered to be an actual cause of dementia.

A few types of dementia, such as Pick's disease (p. 20) and Huntington's disease (p. 21) and rare cases of Alzheimer's disease (p. 4), are known to be inherited, passed on from one generation to the next in the genes. Other types of dementia, including most cases of Alzheimer's disease (p. 6) and also vascular dementia (p. 19), are thought to be caused by a combination of genetic and other factors.

Some types of dementia occur as a feature of some other disease, such as AIDS (p. 22), Parkinson's disease (p. 23) and syphilis.

A person's behaviour can also increase the risk of dementia, even if it does not directly cause it. People who smoke, for example, have an increased risk for vascular dementia and people whose alcohol consumption is excessive may develop alcoholic dementia or Korsakoff's syndrome (p. 25).

Can stress or worry cause dementia?

There is no evidence that stress or worry is responsible for causing dementia. However, stress or worry can lead to forgetfulness and confusion that may sometimes be mistaken for early dementia. It is also true that a diagnosis of dementia is sometimes only made after a period of stress or worry has made the disease more apparent, even though the dementia has in fact been present for some time. Anxiety is a common symptom of depression in older people and the presence of depression can result in severe memory problems that may be mistaken for dementia.

Can aluminium or mercury cause dementia?

Some people do believe that aluminium or mercury can cause dementia. Further research is under way, but at present the arguments do not seem to be very convincing. (See p. 7 and p. 8 for more details.)

My husband has been told that he has some sort of dementia and that he should give up smoking. Can smoking cause dementia?

Smoking is not thought to be a direct cause of dementia, but it can contribute to atherosclerosis (narrowing of the arteries), which often leads to strokes. One form of dementia, called vascular dementia (see p. 19), is caused by strokes, which cause brain damage by cutting of the blood supply to areas of the brain.

Not all doctors would agree that giving up smoking is likely to have much effect on the course of vascular dementia once this disease is already apparent. However, stopping smoking can be recommended on many other grounds.

My father who is 72 has recently had an operation on his bowel. He was a bit forgetful before he went into hospital but now he is home again he is very confused. Might the operation have given him dementia?

Operations do not in themselves cause dementia. They may, however, cause temporary confusion or make pre-existing dementia worse because removal from home to hospital, anaesthetic and even pain-relieving drugs may temporarily increase confusion.

If your father's confusion persists, it is possible that he did have a dementia before the operation, which has been made worse. This sometimes happens after someone has had an anaesthetic. After an anaesthetic older people are vulnerable to having strokes and it is possible that your father has had a small stroke as a consequence of the operation and that this is causing his confusion.

Another possible explanation for your father's confusion is that he has picked up a chest or urinary tract infection. This possibility is less likely if the operation was already some time ago. However, do speak to his doctor about your concerns, as treatment of an infection can sometimes bring about a dramatic improvement.

Can head injuries cause dementia?

People who suffer severe or repeated head injuries are at increased risk of developing dementia. However, the link between head injuries and dementia is not straightforward. It is possible that a head injury may trigger the disease process in susceptible individuals. People who have sustained serious head injuries through boxing are prone to a type of dementia, known as dementia pugilistica, which is similar to Alzheimer's disease.

Types of dementia

What is vascular dementia?

Vascular dementia (also called multi-infarct dementia) is a type of dementia caused by a series of 'mini strokes' (infarcts). It is the second commonest type of dementia, after Alzheimer's disease. Vascular dementia is estimated to account on its own for about one in five dementia cases, and to occur with Alzheimer's disease in another one in five cases.

The mini strokes that cause vascular dementia are often so slight that they cause no immediate symptoms, or they may cause some temporary confusion. However, each stroke destroys a small area of cells in the brain by cutting off its blood supply. The strokes themselves may occur because of high blood pressure, which can cause blood vessels in the brain to burst, or blood clots, which can cause blockages in the vessels supplying blood to the brain. Even though the damage caused by an individual stroke may be slight, the cumulative effect of a number of mini strokes is often sufficient to cause vascular dementia. This type of dementia may also occur if a small stroke affects a crucial part of the brain.

The predominant symptoms of vascular dementia, shared with other dementias, are the loss of short-term memory and the progressive decline in other abilities. However, in vascular dementia, the memory loss is typically much more variable than in Alzheimer's disease. There are also often long periods when a person's memory loss does not seem to be worsening. Then there may be an episode of acute confusion, often in association with a new mini stroke, followed by a step down in the person's memory. Doctors often describe vascular dementia as having a 'step-like' progression.

Other characteristic features of vascular dementia are that people usually have a greater degree of awareness of their disability than is the case with Alzheimer's disease. There is also a relative preservation of personality in vascular dementia and an increased likelihood of problems with unpredictable behaviour.

It seems my mother has Pick's disease. What is this? How does it differ from Alzheimer's disease?

Pick's disease is a rare type of dementia. It shares various similarities with Alzheimer's disease, but also differs from that disease in a number of important respects.

Figure 1: Location of the lobes of the brain

Pick's disease typically develops at an earlier age than Alzheimer's disease, usually in a person's forties or fifties. It is known to have a genetic cause and to run in families more commonly than Alzheimer's disease, but it can also occur when there is no family history of this form of dementia.

The most important difference between Pick's disease and Alzheimer's disease is that the brain tissue changes that occur in Pick's disease typically mainly affect the frontal lobes of the brain. Pick's disease causes marked shrinkage of these lobes while leaving other parts of the brain relatively unaffected. As with Alzheimer's disease, a definite diagnosis of Pick's disease requires a post mortem examination. However, in practice, the diagnosis can often be made from a person's symptoms and signs. If a doctor suspects Pick's disease, he or she will sometimes ask a psychologist to do specific tests which can help the diagnosis.

People with Pick's disease often have what doctors describe as 'frontal lobe symptoms'. This means that they become typically apathetic and withdrawn, and their personality may change. For example, they may become more placid or, occasionally, more aggressive. Some people with Pick's disease also become disinhibited, which can be very difficult for carers. The other cardinal feature of Pick's disease is that people with this form of dementia have problems expressing themselves. This is because the area of the brain which is involved in creating speech (Broca's area in the left frontal lobe) is often affected.

The outlook for people with Pick's disease is similar to that for people with Alzheimer's disease. A progressive decline in abilities will typically lead to death between five and 10 years after diagnosis.

My boyfriend says he doesn't want to get serious with me because there is Huntington's disease in his family. What does this mean?

Huntington's disease, sometimes known as Huntington's chorea, is a relatively rare form of dementia in which mental

H 0, 4 10 /616·831.

deterioration is accompanied by problems in controlling body movements. Huntington's disease is an inherited disease. If your boyfriend's mother or father has the disease, there is a one in two chance that he (and also any of his brothers or sisters) will also develop it.

People at risk of developing Huntington's disease can have genetic counselling and then a genetic test to find out whether or not they have inherited the abnormal gene that will give them the disease. However, it is important to respect a person's wishes if he or she prefers not to find out this information in advance.

Huntington's disease usually becomes apparent when people are in their thirties or forties, although symptoms can start sooner. The illness may begin with either mental or physical symptoms. Progressive loss of memory and concentration, leading to severe dementia, may be accompanied by anxiety, irritability and depression. The movement problems that characterise this disease take the form of involuntary twitching and spasms of the muscles (known as chorea).

There is no specific treatment for Huntington's disease, but drugs do sometimes help the chorea. The illness typically lasts for 10 to 25 years, leading to severe disability and eventual death. As the disease progresses, 24-hour nursing care will inevitably be needed.

Do most people with HIV develop dementia?

Most people with HIV – the virus that leads to AIDS – do not develop dementia. However, there is a possibility that someone infected with HIV may develop subtle memory problems before developing AIDS.

Some people who have AIDS develop severe dementia, often characterised by apathy. This is sometimes known as AIDS-related cognitive impairment. The dementia that occurs with AIDS is sometimes due to a direct effect of the HIV virus on the brain. In other cases, the dementia is due to infections or tumours of the brain that develop because of lowered immunity.

My father has had Parkinson's disease for three years now and seems to be getting quite forgetful. I have heard he may develop dementia – is this true?

It is true that people with Parkinson's disease do have an increased risk of developing dementia. An estimated 15 to 20 per cent of people diagnosed as having Parkinson's disease also have some form of dementia. Some people with Parkinson's disease have been found to have a type of dementia known as Lewy body disease (see the next answer for more information). However, the fact that your father is showing signs of forgetfulness does not mean that he is necessarily developing dementia.

It is possible that your father's memory is working perfectly well but he appears to have a problem because he is slowed up. Even if he does have a memory problem, this may not be due to dementia. For example, people who have Parkinson's disease are often treated with drugs belonging to a drug group known as anticholinergics (see Glossary). These drugs can improve Parkinson's disease but they also sometimes make someone's memory worse. Also, people with Parkinson's disease sometimes become depressed. Depression is a common cause of poor memory, which is sometimes misinterpreted as dementia (see p. 30 for more information).

I thought my husband had Alzheimer's disease but the specialist says it is Lewy body disease. What are the differences? Will the fact that my husband has Lewy body disease affect how I can look after him?

Lewy body disease is a form of dementia that is similar to Alzheimer's disease. It takes its name from abnormal collections of protein, known as Lewy bodies, which occur in the nerve cells of the brain.

Your husband probably has symptoms and signs similar to those of someone with Parkinson's disease, such as having a tremor, being somewhat unsteady on his feet and being rather slowed up. He may also be experiencing visual hallucinations (see p. 87). It is also likely that your husband's condition will vary from day to day, and that on some days he will have a short episode of being very confused, which will then settle. This pattern is typical of Lewy body disease but is not common in Alzheimer's disease.

In terms of care, your husband's needs will be much the same as if he had been found to have Alzheimer's disease rather than Lewy body disease. The main difference is that you may find it more difficult to predict how he is going to feel on a day-to-day basis compared to someone with Alzheimer's disease.

People will Lewy body disease are very sensitive to some tranquillisers known as antipsychotic or neuroleptic drugs (see p. 161) and their use should be avoided if at all possible.

My wife, who is 75, started to lose her memory about 10 years ago and five years ago was diagnosed with Alzheimer's disease. We have both eaten a lot of beef. Do you think she might have CJD not Alzheimer's?

Your wife is very unlikely to have CJD (Creutzfeld Jakob disease). CJD is an extremely rare type of dementia which affects only one in a million people in the UK, whereas Alzheimer's disease affects around one in 10 people of your wife's age. However, the main reason for thinking that your wife is unlikely to have CJD is that her illness has now lasted for a number of years. CJD usually progresses very rapidly and is often fatal within a year.

Many of the early signs of CJD are similar to Alzheimer's disease but there are some differences. People with CJD may become rather withdrawn and forgetful, and soon develop problems in finding the right words and having a conversation. They also become unsteady on their feet and frequently have spasms or jerky movements in their arms and legs.

Over the last few years, there has been a lot of publicity about a possible link between CJD and BSE (bovine spongiform encephalopathy), a similar disease that affects cows. CJD, BSE, and a disease called scrapie in sheep, are all known to be caused by an unusual infectious agent called a prion. It is thought that a few cases of CJD that have occurred recently in young people may be linked to eating beef from cows infected with BSE. However, these young people appear to have contracted a distinctive new form of CJD. No link has been found between beef eating and the more usual form of CJD, which typically develops in late middle age. (The Alzheimer's Disease Society has a CJD Support Network: see Appendix 1.)

Might dementia be due to a brain tumour?

Brain tumours are a rare cause of dementia. One type of slow-growing brain tumour, known as a meningioma, some-times causes symptoms of dementia. Most brain tumours cause other kinds of symptoms, such as headaches, loss of limb function, visual disturbance and loss of balance. In some cases, removal of a meningioma may result in recovery from the dementia.

Can water on the brain cause dementia?

One type of dementia, known as normal pressure hydro-cephalus is due not to water but to an excess of cerebrospinal fluid in the brain. Early symptoms of this type of dementia include incontinence of urine and problems with walking. If your doctor suspects this type of dementia, he or she may order a brain scan to confirm the diagnosis. (Also see p. 165.)

Does drinking too much alcohol cause dementia?

People who drink too much alcohol do seem to be at risk of developing problems with their memory. Some have a specific problem of loss of short-term memory (see p. 11), known as Korsakoff's syndrome, which develops because of vitamin B_1 (thiamine) deficiency. Others develop a wider range of problems that resemble Alzheimer's disease. Drinking moderate amounts of alcohol is probably safe.

Can hormone deficiencies cause dementia?

Underactivity of the thyroid gland can result in a condition called hypothyroidism, of which dementia can be a symptom. People with hypothyroidism typically gain weight and develop a hoarse voice, dry skin and thinning hair. Hypothyroidism can be simply treated with replacement thyroid hormones. Some other hormone deficiencies are rare causes of dementia.

Can dietary deficiencies cause dementia? My wife has been a vegetarian for many years and now has dementia. Could her diet be to blame?

It is true that dietary deficiencies are a rare cause of dementia. However, it is very unlikely that your wife's dementia has been caused by her vegetarianism. Your wife is much more likely to be suffering from one of the more common types of dementia, such as Alzheimer's disease.

Deficiencies of some vitamins, such as vitamin B_{12} or B_1 (thiamine), have been implicated as rare causes of dementia. These vitamins are present in a wide range of foods and can be stored by the body for long periods. It is uncommon for anyone to develop a deficiency of either of these vitamins.

People who drink excessive amounts of alcohol over a long period of time sometimes develop a deficiency of vitamin B_1, leading to Korsakoff's syndrome. People on a vegan diet, which excludes not only meat but also eggs and milk, may need supplementary vitamin B_{12}.

A few people develop a deficiency of vitamin B_{12} because their bodies do not absorb this vitamin properly. This is usually because of pernicious anaemia due to either a rare stomach problem, known as intrinsic factor deficiency, or to previous surgery to the bowel.

Although dementia due to vitamin deficiency is rare, your wife's doctor will probably have already carried out a blood test to exclude this possibility. In cases where a vitamin B_{12} deficiency is found, the usual treatment is to give the vitamin by injection every three months.

3

Getting a diagnosis

Introduction

Alzheimer's disease and other dementias usually develop slowly and people may have been ill for some time before the diagnosis is thought of. Getting a diagnosis is important. If someone is diagnosed as having Alzheimer's disease or another dementia, then carers are better able to plan for the future and will be more prepared for what will happen. Although there is no specific test for Alzheimer's disease, various tests and investigations can help show whether or not someone has the disease. This chapter explains some of the ways doctors try and diagnose Alzheimer's disease and some of the tests and investigations that may be used.

The need for diagnosis

Why is diagnosis so important?

A proper medical diagnosis is needed whenever anyone develops dementia-like symptoms and does not appear to be getting any better. Diagnosis is important because:
- it can rule out the possibility that the symptoms have a different, more easily treatable cause;
- it allows family members, friends, and, whenever possible, sufferers themselves to make plans for the future if Alzheimer's disease or another dementia is diagnosed;
- it leads to the appropriate care and treatment of a person with Alzheimer's disease or another dementia.

I'm not sure, but I think my wife may be developing Alzheimer's disease. I have heard there is no cure, so is it necessary to involve the doctor?

You should definitely involve the doctor as soon as possible if you suspect that your wife may be developing Alzheimer's disease. There are several important reasons.

First, your wife may have a condition that looks like Alzheimer's disease, but which is treatable. Examples include depression (see p. 30), under-activity of the thyroid gland (see p. 26) or Parkinson's disease (see p. 23). Infections or constipation can also cause temporary confusion, as can some medicines, such as strong painkillers, blood pressure treatment or tranquillisers. Your wife's doctor will want to examine your wife and probably do some blood tests before coming to a diagnosis of dementia.

A second important reason to get a diagnosis is that this will help you and your wife to make plans for the future. For example, if it is found that your wife does have Alzheimer's disease, you should consider organising an Enduring Power of Attorney (see p. 134) while she is still able to do this. You will also be able to investigate the various types of help that may be available (see Chapter 9). It may also be necessary to discourage your wife from driving.

Third, drug treatments that may help to decrease the symptoms of confusion are becoming available (see p. 156) and are more likely to help if started early in the disease.

Is there any point in telling the difference between Alzheimer's disease and vascular dementia?

It can be difficult to determine whether someone is suffering from Alzheimer's disease, vascular dementia (see p. 19) or a mixture of the two. However, it is worth trying to tell the difference because this may affect how someone can best be looked after.

Alzheimer's disease and vascular dementia together account for by far the greater majority of cases of dementia in the United Kingdom. (About 50 per cent of dementia cases are thought to be due to Alzheimer's disease alone, 20 per cent to vascular dementia alone, and 20 per cent to both causes.) If there is a history of high blood pressure or stroke, or if a CT scan shows evidence of strokes in the brain, it is likely that a person is suffering from vascular dementia. This type of dementia is also characterised by a more step-like progression, rather than the steadier decline typical of Alzheimer's disease.

If someone has vascular dementia, then the doctor may want to prescribe aspirin or other drugs to thin the blood and try to prevent further strokes. If someone has Alzheimer's disease, especially if the disease is at an early stage, then they may be helped by one of the new anticholinesterase drugs (see p. 156). Other treatments for memory impairment may also become available in future.

My wife, who has Alzheimer's disease, seems to be very withdrawn and increasingly forgetful. Is this due to the disease, or might she also be suffering from depression? Can the doctor do anything to help?

When someone has Alzheimer's disease or another dementia, it can be very difficult to decide if they are suffering from depression as well. If you are worried that your wife may be depressed, do tell her doctor.

Depression in someone with dementia may occur independently of the dementia, or it may result from the dementia itself. Moodiness, anxiety, fear and puzzlement are all understandable emotions in people with dementia, especially early in the illness when they still have some awareness of their failing capacities. Someone in your wife's position will also be sensitive to the moods of the people around her. If there is tension at home it is likely she will respond to it, although not necessarily in a clear or appropriate way. If people with dementia become depressed, they often cannot express these feelings in words. However, they may become slow and withdrawn and appear more confused and forgetful. They may also lose their appetite, causing loss of weight.

It is certainly important to identify depression in someone with dementia, because treating the depression (see p. 163) can help them feel better and make a significant contribution towards enabling them to make the best use of their failing mental abilities.

Seeking a diagnosis

My husband has recently been showing disturbing signs of memory loss but won't see a doctor. Can you advise me?

Reluctance on the part of someone with memory problems to seek medical advice is common and understandable. Your husband may have no idea that anything is wrong, or alternatively he may fear that there is a problem but hope that it will 'go away'.

If the difficulties have arisen quite suddenly – within weeks rather than months – then seeking a medical opinion is a matter of urgency. If the loss of memory has been more gradual, then the need for your husband to see a doctor is slightly less urgent. If at all possible, enlist your GP's help. He or she may well have developed a diplomatic way of overcoming this sort of problem. One possibility is for you to suggest to your husband that both of you ought to attend the doctor's surgery for a routine health check.

If for any reason your GP can't help, you could speak to the Alzheimer's Disease Society (see Appendix 1) about the possibility of getting in touch directly with the psychiatric service that deals with problems of the elderly in your area.

Don't give up trying to persuade your husband to see a doctor – patience and perseverance generally pays. Your husband's mood and willingness to accept help may well vary from day to day. He may eventually agree on the grounds of saving you from worry.

When you do succeed in arranging for your husband to see a doctor, be prepared. Take time beforehand to draw up a written list of the problems, and of any questions you would like to be answered. If you are present when your husband is being interviewed, try not to interrupt or to prompt him. It is important for the doctor to be able to make his or her own independent assessment of your husband's condition. However, do ensure that you also have a time in which you can talk to the doctor without interruption.

I am sure my husband is starting with Alzheimer's disease. But every time I take him to our GP he puts on a show and convinces the doctor he is all right. Now the doctor has prescribed me tranquillisers! What can I do?

If you are really worried, you should seek further advice. It can sometimes be difficult to diagnose Alzheimer's disease in its early stages.

It is possible that you are right and your husband does have early Alzheimer's disease. Sometimes people can appear very convincing in the early stages of the disease, and the doctor may have been misled by this. On the other hand, it is also possible that your husband does not have Alzheimer's disease. Many people become more forgetful as they get get older, without this amounting to Alzheimer's disease or progressing very much.

Before visiting the doctor again, it would probably be worth keeping a diary of your husband's symptoms. Nearly everyone forgets to say important things when they are sitting in front of the doctor, so writing them down first, either to read yourself or to show to the doctor, can be very helpful. If your GP has other partners in the practice, you could try speaking to one of them. You could also ask for your husband to be referred to a specialist for a second opinion.

If you feel that the relationship with your doctor has broken down irretrievably, then you are entitled to move to a different practice. Your local Public Library will have a list of doctors' practices in your area.

My father is seventy and clearly has a problem with his memory. He is Chairman of a Board of Directors and is quite unaware that he has a problem. I am very worried he will make a fool of himself. What can I do?

This is a very difficult situation. You need to work out first how bad the memory problem is. Is it that your father just has a problem in remembering names, or does he show much more inappropriate behaviour than this? If his behaviour is inappropriate, is this because of his memory problem or is it related to his mood? Sometimes depression can cause symptoms similar to those of dementia. In any event, you should probably try to persuade your father to see his doctor. If that is not possible, because he sees no reason to go, then it might be useful for you to talk to his doctor yourself.

If your father does not recognise that he has a problem, you may feel the need to talk to someone at his work. This will obviously be easier if you know any of his colleagues personally. However, before taking this possibly drastic step, which could lead to his removal from the Board, you must ask yourself how much all this really matters. It may be reasonable to wait until one of his colleagues notices your father's difficulties and then approaches either you or your father's doctor. On the other hand, if your father's work holds considerable responsibility and affects the lives of other people, you may need to take the initiative and talk to one of his colleagues sooner rather than later.

The process of diagnosis

How is Alzheimer's disease usually diagnosed?

A diagnosis of Alzheimer's disease is usually made on the basis of a patient's symptoms and mental abilities. To obtain as much information as possible, the doctor will undertake a process known as 'history taking', during which he or she will talk to the patient, and probably also to someone else who knows the patient well, such as a family member or friend. There may also be a more formal assessment of a patient's physical and mental condition and needs (see p. 108).

It is often difficult to make a conclusive diagnosis of Alzheimer's disease. Various other illnesses, such as depression (see p. 30), a thyroid problem (p. 26), a vitamin deficiency (p. 26) or Parkinson's disease (p. 23), can cause similar symptoms. A full physical examination, and various tests, including blood tests (see p. 38) and perhaps a brain scan (see p. 40), can help rule out some of the other possibilities. If tests fail to show any other reason for a person's symptoms, a doctor will often make a diagnosis of Alzheimer's disease. Sometimes, the diagnosis is made only after observing how a patient's condition develops over a period of several months.

Is there a quick test for Alzheimer's disease? I think I read something about one in a magazine.

There is no simple, single, straightforward test for Alzheimer's disease. There have been some press reports about quick tests for Alzheimer's disease, but no such test is available at the present time.

Tests of various kinds, including blood tests (see p. 38) and brain scans (see p. 40), can help doctors to rule out other possible causes of symptoms that resemble those of Alzheimer's disease. In rare cases, a genetic test (see p. 39) will help confirm the diagnosis.

An absolutely certain diagnosis of Alzheimer's disease usually requires a post mortem examination (see p. 3). In practice, however, such examinations are rarely performed.

I am going to see the doctor because I think my mother may have Alzheimer's disease as she is so forgetful. What sort of things will the doctor want to know?

The doctor will want to know as much as possible about your mother's problem. You may find it useful to make some notes before the appointment. Try to remember when you first noticed your mother's forgetfulness. Also think about how it has progressed. Did the problem occur suddenly, or has it developed gradually over a period of time?

Unless the doctor already knows your mother quite well, he or she will want to ask you some details about about your mother's life. For example, the type of work she does or did, the sort of person she is and what things she likes doing. The doctor might also want to ask you about aspects of your mother's medical history, including information about past illnesses and operations, and whether anyone else in the family has ever suffered from Alzheimer's disease.

The GP was unable to decide whether my wife has Alzheimer's disease and is making arrangements for her to see a specialist. What will this involve?

The exact procedure for involving a specialist in a possible case of Alzheimer's disease varies, depending on the GP and on which hospital consultant is approached. All consultants will want to ask about the patient's symptoms, in addition to the questions already asked by the GP.

Many consultants believe a first assessment is best done in the patient's home. Your GP will advise you if this is to happen in your wife's case. A consultant who visits a patient at home will be able to pick up additional clues about the patient's condition and will be able to assess how well or badly the patient is coping in his or her home.

Other consultants prefer to see each patient, with a family member or friend, in a day hospital or clinic. You will be sent appointment details for your wife in due course if you have not already received them. The advantages of this approach are that it may be easier to conduct a thorough examination of the patient, that various investigations and tests can be carried out on the same day, and that a range of other professionals are on hand to help with the assessment.

If your wife is found to have Alzheimer's disease or one of the other dementias, a thorough assessment should extend beyond purely medical matters. It may cover, for example, how well she is able to cope in the home setting, your financial circumstances and whether Social Services are involved. A medical assessment is part of the 'needs assessment' (see p. 108) that determines the types of community care that may be available (see Chapter 9: Getting help).

We went to the doctor because my husband is getting very forgetful. Now we have an appointment for a memory clinic. What is a memory clinic?

Different memory clinics work in different ways. The people who work there may include doctors, nurses, psychologists, occupational therapists and social workers. So it is difficult to generalise about the ways they work. However, if you attend a memory clinic you can expect that a doctor at the clinic will want to hear an account of the illness, from your husband and also from yourself. A psychologist may give your husband a special memory test (see below). An occupational therapist may assess your husband's abilities to manage around the home. Social workers will be able to advise you on how to deal with some of the implications of a diagnosis of Alzheimer's disease.

Sometimes, memory clinics are run by doctors who are conducting trials into drugs that might prevent further memory problems. It is worth remembering that people with memory problems often need a wide range of assessment and that they need to be in touch with local Social Services. So if your husband has been referred to a memory clinic that is some distance away, it is important that you and he are not cut off from local services. You should discuss this with your husband's GP and with Social Services.

When the doctor told me that my wife has Alzheimer's disease I was so shocked that I didn't take in everything he said. What should I do?

This is quite common. Don't be embarrassed about making an appointment to talk to the doctor again. It is important that you have a discussion about what your needs are, what sort of help is possible and what to expect in the future. It is also important that you try to ensure that there is some ongoing follow-up of both you and your wife, as the situation is inevitably going to change as time goes on.

Memory tests

My wife was visited by a psychiatrist and then a few weeks later by a community psychiatric nurse. Both did a test which I think was called the Mental State Examination. What is this and why do they do it, as it seems to distress my wife?

The Mini Mental State Examination is one of a number of screening tests for dementia. It takes about five to six minutes to administer and involves asking people a set of questions to test their memory, orientation as regards to time and place, understanding and language ability. People taking the test are also asked to write a sentence and to copy a drawing.

The Mini Mental State Examination is commonly used by professionals caring for people with dementia. It is not a diagnostic test as the information it gives is not sufficient to allow a diagnosis of Alzheimer's disease or another dementia to be made. People can score low on the test for a number of different reasons. The test can, however, be useful for monitoring people's mental abilities in the early stages of dementia. Occasionally, people do get upset when they are asked apparently simple questions that they cannot answer or get wrong. If this happens it may be better to leave things alone and return to the test later.

My partner has to see a psychologist next week for some kind of memory test. Can you explain why he needs to go and what will be involved?

Making a diagnosis of dementia can be quite difficult, especially when the illness is in its early stages. Furthermore, some people may complain of poor memory that is not obvious when the doctor first sees them. It is in these sort of circumstances that a doctor may decide to refer a patient to a clinical psychologist or another doctor in order to have a more extensive set of memory tests.

Two commonly used tests are known as the Wechsler Adult Intelligence Scale and the Cambridge Cognitive Test (CAMCOG). Both of these tests are divided into a number of different sections and will test a variety of things, including the ability to learn new things and the ability to comprehend arithmetic and vocabulary. Such tests also usually include an assessment of physical skills, such as drawing and copying.

It is important to remember that these tests alone cannot provide a diagnosis of dementia. Your partner's scores will be compared to what would be expected for a person of the same age and background, and even then can do no more than provide an indication of whether there is a problem.

Blood tests

The doctor recently did some blood tests on my wife, but didn't tell me what they were for. Is there a blood test for Alzheimer's disease?

Most cases of Alzheimer's disease cannot be diagnosed by a blood test. However, any person with symptoms that might be due to a dementia such as Alzheimer's disease is likely to be given various blood tests to make sure the symptoms don't have a treatable cause.

The blood tests would normally include a check of kidney and liver function, thyroid gland activity and vitamin levels in the blood. Sometimes, the doctor may check for the presence of syphilis or the HIV virus. The genetic test (see p. 39) for the rare inherited cases of Alzheimer's disease (see p. 4) takes the form of a blood test.

Do not be afraid to ask the doctor about any tests that he or she might perform on your wife.

My partner, a man of forty, is becoming very forgetful. His doctor wants him to have an HIV test. I am sure that my partner has been faithful and that he does not have HIV. Is the test really necessary?

Any type of dementia at the age of 40 is uncommon and requires thorough investigation. Infection with HIV (human immunodeficiency virus) is one possible cause of dementia in younger people. This virus, which is associated with AIDS (acquired immune deficiency syndrome), can enter the brain and cause problems of its own accord, or it can result in other disorders affecting the brain, such as fungal infections.

Some people with HIV infection or AIDS do develop a form of dementia.

Some doctors will recommend an HIV test only if they think that a patient is at particular risk of HIV infection, for example, a gay man, someone who shares needles when injecting drugs, or someone who has received blood or blood products abroad. Other doctors will recommend an HIV test simply because they want to make sure they have considered every possible cause of dementia, especially in a younger person like your partner. All people who are considering having an HIV test should first receive counselling.

If an HIV test is performed and turns out to be positive, it means that appropriate treatment can be given without delay. Drugs can be prescribed to slow down the progress of AIDS. Also, knowing that someone is HIV positive enables doctors to keep a look out for other conditions associated with AIDs, such as fungal infections, and to treat these early.

It is also useful for doctors to know that a younger patient with dementia is HIV negative. Having ruled out HIV as a possible cause of the dementia, they can move on to more extensive investigations to try and find out the actual cause.

Genetic test

My grandmother, father and uncle all developed Alzheimer's disease around age fifty. It seems our family may have a rare inherited form of the disease. I've been offered a genetic test, but don't know whether to have it. What are the advantages and disadvantages?

This is a complex question and it is better to talk the issues through with a trained counsellor and a doctor who specialises in genetic diseases. Don't be hurried into a decision.

If you do have the test, which is a simple blood test, it will show whether or not you are carrying the gene that has caused Alzheimer's disease in your family. Because your father had the gene, you have a one in two chance of having inherited it. If you do have the gene, you will almost certainly develop Alzheimer's disease at around the same age as the other members of your family. If you don't have the gene, then this is very unlikely.

The disadvantages of the test are that if it shows that you do have the gene you may have difficulty getting life insurance, mortgages or even a job if you declare that you have had it. You may also find it hard to cope with the knowledge that you will develop a disease for which there is no cure. On the other hand, you may prefer to know what to expect, so that you can plan your life accordingly. You may also be wondering about having children and want to know if you are at risk of passing on the gene to them.

Brain scans

My doctor has diagnosed my mother as having Alzheimer's disease, but has not done a brain scan. Isn't a brain scan necessary in every case?

No. In fact the usual type of brain scan (a CT scan, see p. 41) is of limited use in diagnosing Alzheimer's disease and most other dementias. All the brain scan is likely to show is some shrinkage of the brain, but this can occur in people who do not have dementia. Also, an entirely normal scan does not rule out the possibility of dementia.

The main reasons for doing a brain scan are if a patient's symptoms are not typical, or if the doctor suspects a brain tumour. A brain tumour (see p. 25) is a very rare cause of dementia, and other symptoms and findings when the doctor examines the patient would be likely to suggest this diagnosis. Brain scans can also point to whether someone is suffering from vascular dementia (see p. 19) rather than Alzheimer's disease, but again this information is often apparent from a person's medical history.

What is the difference between a CT scan and a CAT scan?

There is no difference. The terms CT scan and CAT scan are both abbreviations for Computerised Axial Tomography. (See the next answer for details).

My wife is having a CT scan of her brain. What does this involve?

A CT scan is a way of taking pictures of the brain using X-rays and a computer. The result is a series of computer-generated pictures that show slices of the brain. CT scans are useful for diagnosing strokes and tumours. They may also show changes, such as thinning of the brain tissue, that occur in people with Alzheimer's disease. CT scans can also help doctors to distinguish between vascular dementia (see p. 19) and Alzheimer's disease.

A CT scan will normally be performed on an out-patient basis, with the scan itself taking between 15 and 30 minutes. Some people find the procedure rather disturbing and may not be able to stay still long enough. If a scan is considered to be absolutely necessary for someone who is likely to become agitated, then he or she may be given a light sedative. An injection, containing a harmless dye, may be given to help show the brain more clearly.

The CT scanner looks a bit like a very large front-loading washing machine. It may be in a room with a lot of equip-ment and may look a little daunting at first. Your wife will be asked to lie on a narrow bed with her head near the scanner entrance. The scan will be performed by a radiographer, who will operate the controls from an adjacent room and will watch your wife through a large window. The bed on which your wife is lying will move into the scanner, and a series of X-rays will be taken. There is a little noise.

At the end, there will be a series of about 20 pictures showing your wife's brain from top to bottom. If your wife was given a sedative you will have to wait for the effects to wear off. Otherwise, you will be able to go home immediately after the scan. The radiographer will not be able to give you any results. These will take a few days because the films from the scan will need to be examined closely.

What is an MRI scan? Is it better than a CT scan?

MRI stands for Magnetic Resonance Imaging. Like CT scans, MRI scans use a computer to create pictures of slices through the brain. But unlike CT scans, MRI scans do not use X-rays to obtain the image. Instead, they use radio signals produced by the body in response to the effects of a very strong magnet contained within the scanner.

MRI scans show more detail than CT scans, but they take longer to do, and are more expensive. Sometimes a doctor will ask for an MRI scan if the CT scan doesn't show enough information.

Like CT scanners, MRI scanners look like large washing machines: the hole in the middle is the scanner entrance. MRI scans are quite noisy, and can take up to an hour to do. It is essential that the person having the scan remains very still throughout, and this can cause some discomfort.

I took my partner to see a specialist and he ordered a SPECT scan. What is this?

SPECT stands for Single Photon Emission Computerised Tomography. This type of scan, unlike a CT scan or an MRI scan, looks at blood flow through the brain, rather than at the structure of the brain. Research suggests that the information provided by a SPECT scan may help in confirming the diagnosis of dementia in some cases.

A SPECT scan is very simple. The person to be scanned is first given an injection of a very mild radioactive substance, which is quite safe. This substance (a radionuclide) travels in the blood to the brain. The person then has to sit still while the scanner, which looks like a rotating hair dryer, takes pictures of the brain. The result is a series of computer-generated pictures of slices of the brain. These slices are like a map. They show variations in the amount of radionuclide that is taken up by the brain. This in turn shows how well the blood is flowing to different areas within the brain.

Talking about the diagnosis

My wife has just been diagnosed with Alzheimer's disease, but she doesn't know this yet. Should I tell her and, if so, how?

In general, research suggests that most people prefer to be told what is wrong with them. There is also an increasingly common belief that all people, including those with dementia, have a right to know their diagnosis, whatever it might be. Whether or not you agree with this, or whether or not you believe that your wife will benefit from being told her diagnosis, may depend on individual circumstances. You probably know your wife better than anyone, which may help you to decide how she is likely to respond to the information. Also, if your wife is already very confused, it may not be helpful to tell her. On the other hand, you may find that, even though she is confused, she understands more than you think she does and will be helped by being told.

If you think your wife would like to know, but you are unhappy about telling her yourself, you can ask the doctor to tell her while you are with her. A surprising number of people will accept being told sensitively by a doctor that they clearly have a problem with their memory and that they will require help to cope with it. Others will want to know the actual diagnosis so that they can help make plans for the future while they are still able to do so.

If you decide to tell your wife yourself, choose a quiet moment when you are not likely to be interrupted. Sit down close to her, perhaps touching her arm or holding her hand. Watch her carefully as you speak and take her reactions into account as you proceed. Try to assess how much information she is ready to receive. Talking about the diagnosis will be emotionally very difficult, but it could help you both to share this information.

It is important in this situation to try to tell the truth and to avoid saying anything that is misleading. Don't tell her that it is simply her age or that she has nothing to worry about. You may decide that it is not helpful in your wife's case to 'label' the illness as Alzheimer's disease, but even so you should try not to withhold information if she asks you a direct question. Trust is essential when caring for someone with Alzheimer's disease, and once trust is broken it is hard to restore.

After your wife has been told the diagnosis, you may find that she is unable to face up to the reality of the disease. She may deny strongly and persistently that there is a problem. If this is the case, try to avoid getting drawn into an argument or confrontation with her. The denial may be a device to give her time to come to terms with the diagnosis.

Provided that the diagnosis is made in the early stages of the disease, it is quite possible that your wife will be able to take an active part in the legal and financial planning which should take place as soon as possible after the diagnosis has been made (see Chapter 11 for details). This planning process may in itself help everyone concerned to come to terms with what the disease entails.

My husband, who has Alzheimer's disease, gets upset when he forgets things. Should I remind him about his diagnosis, so that he can understand what is happening to him?

Some people in the early stages of Alzheimer's disease seem to appreciate that their memory is failing. Gently reminding them of the reason for this may help them feel less pressured and so reduce stress. However, as time goes on, people who have Alzheimer's disease become generally unaware of their problems. Reminding someone with more advanced

Alzheimer's disease that their memory is failing is unlikely to help them to understand their condition and may add to their distress.

My mother, who lives with us, has been diagnosed with Alzheimer's disease. I have been so worried about her that I have not been able to work out what to tell my children. They realise there is something wrong with their grandmother. What should I say?

Children are very resilient and generally respond well to being told the truth. Explain the facts to them as clearly as you can, and give them plenty of opportunity to ask questions. You should have this conversation with them as soon as possible because they may be blaming themselves for their grandmother's strange behaviour. Finding out that it is due to an illness is likely to be a relief to them.

This is a difficult time for all of you. The best way of helping your children to cope with it is to give them plenty of explanations, reassurance, hugs and love. The Alzheimer's Disease Society (address in Appendix 1) has produced a booklet entitled 'It's Me Grandma! It's Me!' to help children in this situation. There is also a leaflet for teenagers.

4
Practical care day to day

Introduction

Activities such as as dressing, washing, going to the toilet, eating and sleeping are a normal part of everyday life. However, even these routine tasks become increasingly difficult for people with Alzheimer's disease to perform on their own. This chapter provides some useful guidelines as to how carers might be able to help the people they are looking after to live as well and as independently as possible.

The amount of help that a carer needs to give will obviously change over time.

General questions

My father who has Alzheimer's disease is coming to live with me and my family. Can you give me any tips as I fear he is going to be difficult to look after?

Living with and caring for a person with Alzheimer's disease can be very difficult at times. The following tips have been recommended by other carers:
- Try to establish a routine.
- Allow your father some independence.
- Maintain his dignity.
- Avoid confrontation whenever possible.
- Keep tasks simple.
- Maintain a sense of humour.
- Make sure your home is as safe as possible.
- Encourage your father to take exercise.
- Help make the best of your father's existing abilities.
- Remember problems are due to the disease not the person.
- At all times be flexible because Alzheimer's disease is a progressive illness and you are going to have to adapt with the changes that occur as time goes on.

My husband has recently been diagnosed as having Alzheimer's disease. I am in my early seventies and still very fit. How long am I likely to be able to carry on looking after him in our home?

The answer to this question will depend on the rate at which your husband's illness progresses, on your own on-going state of health, and on how much support you can get from family, friends and outside agencies. (See Chapter 9 for information on getting help.) Even with support, you are unlikely to be able to manage your husband at home in the later stages of his illness. It is not really possible to predict in advance how long it will be before this point is reached.

Is my wife with dementia able to do less and less for herself because I am doing more and more for her?

Your wife is able to do less and less because dementia is a progressive condition. This means that her abilities will inevitably decline with time. You will need to do more and more for her as time goes on, but if you do too much for her too soon her abilities will decline more rapidly.

It is important to recognise the things that your wife can still do for herself and to allow her to do these even though she may take a long time to do them. If you disregard what she is still capable of, and do everything for her, she will quickly lose the functions that she still has. Try to be patient and to take over from her only the things that she really can no longer manage. The progressive nature of the disease means that the situation will continue to change. You will be able to respond best to your wife's changing needs if you observe her carefully and can be flexible in your attitudes.

My mother has Alzheimer's disease. She also has painful-looking leg ulcers. She doesn't complain about them. Can people with dementia feel pain?

It can be quite difficult to know whether or not someone with Alzheimer's disease or another dementia is experiencing pain. This is particularly true later in the illness, when people are not only unable to tell you that they are in pain, but when even their normal responses to pain can be difficult to interpret.

Recognising that someone is in pain is less of a problem earlier in the illness, particularly if you are looking after someone you have known for a long time. You will usually be able to tell that something is wrong from the way that the person behaves. For example, he or she may become restless, sleep badly or not want to eat. However, even though you may recognise that the person is in pain, you will not be able to rely on him or her to tell you where the pain is or how severe it may be. You (or the doctor) will have to work this out from what you know about the person.

In general, it is best to assume that a procedure that would normally be painful – such as having a leg ulcer dressed – would be equally painful for someone who has dementia, even though they cannot tell you about it.

Dressing

I want my husband, who has dementia, to carry on dressing himself for as long as possible. However, he is finding it increasingly difficult. Can you suggest how I might be able to make dressing easier for him?

You are right to continue to encourage your husband to dress himself, as this will help him to retain his sense of independence and self-esteem.

One way of helping your husband to continue to dress himself is to make sure that he always has plenty of time. Provided that the room is warm, it does not matter if dressing takes a while. It might also help him to manage better if you lay his clothes out for him in the order he needs to put them on. Later in the illness, you will probably need to hand his clothes to him one at a time, and give instructions as to how to put them on.

Some clothes are easier to put on than others. Neck openings should be a good size. Raglan or drop sleeves are easier than tight sleeves. Slip-on shoes are useful. Clothes with elasticated openings or Velcro fastenings are simpler than clothes fastened with buttons. Some people find t-shirts and track suits are an excellent substitute for ordinary shirts, trousers and jackets. However, if your husband has been used to wearing more traditional clothing in the past, he may not like the change. If at all possible, do try to involve him in choosing what he is going to wear each day.

I'm having real problems persuading my mother not to wear the same clothes for days on end. She used to be really smart but now she often looks unkempt. She gets so upset if I say anything. Can you advise?

Your mother probably no longer recognises the need to change her clothes nor knows which ones are clean and which need washing. One possible way to help might be to encourage her to have a bath and then take this opportunity to remove the clothes that need washing and to lay out a clean set for her. If you do this, she will probably not notice what you have done and you will not be hurting her feelings.

Personal hygiene

Is it common for people with Alzheimer's disease to hate having their faces washed? My wife does not mind having a bath, but protests at having her face washed. Does it matter?

This is not especially common. What has probably happened is that your wife no longer understands the need to wash her face. She may also find it undignified to have someone else wash her face for her. Of course, it does not really matter if her face is not washed. It certainly is not worth having a battle about this.

You could try buying a new soft and pretty flannel. Then try to make face washing fun by getting your wife to wash your face with it before she either lets you wash her face or washes her own face.

My husband is always washing his hands. He seems to

forget he's just done it. **The main problem is that he keeps leaving the taps running. Several times recently the bathroom has been flooded. Can you advise?**

Various tap adaptations are available. Some will cause water to flow only when someone's hands are under them. Others have an automatic cut off after a certain quantity of water has been run, or after a set time. Your local water company should be able to provide a catalogue. These adaptations may seem expensive, but if you have metered water will probable save you money as well as much mopping up. If you can't afford the adaptation, it may be worth trying your local Social Services or the caring fund of your local Alzheimer's Disease Society branch. An alternative approach, which you have probably tried already, is to find other activities for your husband that may distract him from the repetitive washing activity.

How can I make it safer to give my mother a bath?

Bath time can be dangerous, especially for elderly frail people with dementia. Bathrooms are slippery places, and it can be very difficult to lift someone when they are wet. Use non-slip mats in the bath and on the bathroom floor. To prevent scalding, always put cold water into the bath before adding hot.

You may also need special rails or a bath seat (a device that rests in the bath for a person to sit on). Speak to your mother's doctor or Social Services about obtaining these aids. An occupational therapist can then visit your home to assess your mother's particular needs. It may also be possible to arrange for a care assistant or nurse (see p. 115) to come and give your mother a bath.

My husband, who has Alzheimer's, is increasingly reluctant to take a bath and his personal hygiene is suffering as a result. Can you advise me please?

The whole question of bathing often requires tact and diplomacy. If reminders of the need to bath are no longer effective, then establishing a regular routine will help him to carry out the tasks involved. When his motivation slips, try to ensure that he has a regular event for which it is worth being well groomed, for example, going to the day centre or a visit to a friend or the pub.

Lots of praise and encouragement when he is freshly bathed and dressed is far more valuable than constant criticism about his cleanliness. If your husband is not able to carry out the task of bathing alone, try not to take over more than is absolutely necessary. He may be able to do everything needed to have a bath but might need help to do it in the right order.

It is possible that your husband may respond favourably to being given a degree of choice over bathing. For example, you could ask him whether he wants a bath first thing in the morning or last thing at night. Alternatively, he might accept being told that a warm bath has been run for him as he 'usually has one before bed'. Ensure that the bathroom is warm and minimise any impression that bathing is a chore.

Some older people never or rarely bath, preferring a good strip-down wash. If this has been your husband's preference in the past, it is better to build on this rather than trying to impose a new system.

When I am helping my elderly father, who has Alzheimer's disease, to undress or take a bath, he often shouts 'rape' and tries to push me away.

For many people, undressing and bathing have always been private functions, and it is quite possible that this is what your father believes. He may also find it very odd that he now has to have help with these things. It is also possible that he no longer recognises you and may see you as a stranger invading his privacy.

If your father becomes agitated when you try to bath him, the best thing to do is to abandon the attempt for another time. If the problem continues, it might be worth asking for a nurse to come in and bath him. Alternatively, it might be possible, if your father goes to a day centre, to arrange for him to be given a bath while he is there.

Is it common for people with Alzheimer's disease to become incontinent? Is their incontinence caused mainly by confusion, or are there other causes?

Many people with Alzheimer's disease are occasionally incontinent, especially of urine. Often, confusion is the main cause, but there are other possibilities to be aware of. It is sensible to consult the doctor if someone becomes incontinent, because treatment of the cause may be possible.

If incontinence of urine comes on suddenly, or if the urine has an unpleasant smell or is dark in colour, the problem may be a bladder infection. It should be possible for a doctor to treat such an infection with drugs. Other treatable causes of incontinence of urine include enlargement of the prostate gland in men, and severe constipation, both of which can interfere with the normal flow of urine. Severe constipation can also cause incontinence of faeces, when semi-solid faecal matter leaks around an impacted faecal mass.

The use of certain medicines can also contribute to incontinence. Sedatives and tranquillisers, for example, often reduce the sensation of needing to pass urine and also slow down the instinct to get to the toilet. Diuretics (water pills), which may be needed to treat another problem, may make incontinence more likely by increasing urine production.

My husband, diagnosed with Alzheimer's disease, has begun to wet the bed. What can I do?

If you have not already done so, speak to your husband's GP as the incontinence may be treatable, at least to some extent (see the previous answer). If your husband's bed-wetting is due mainly to increased confusion, then there are a number of practical steps that you can take to reduce the problem.

Try to ensure that he does not have large drinks last thing at night. Also cut down on tea and coffee, which increase

urine output by their diuretic action. Encourage your husband to go to the toilet before he goes to bed. You may find it
helpful to wake him once or twice during the night for a
toilet visit. Also consider whether the toilet is near enough
to the bedroom. Older people may have no time to waste
looking for the toilet. Make sure he is confident in finding
the toilet and managing the door.

You could also consider the use of a commode or bed bottle.
A waterproof mattress cover would be useful. The district
nurse should be able to advise you and to loan you appropriate equipment. He or she should also know about other
possible sources of local help, such as continence advice and
laundry services.

**I'm at the end of my tether. My wife has Alzheimer's
disease. She isn't too bad, but she keeps wetting herself. Now I'm afraid to take her out. What can I do?**

First check with your wife's doctor that her incontinence does
not have a treatable cause (see p. 53), such as a bladder
infection. If no treatable cause for the incontinence is found,
then the following practical steps may help.

Try to remind your wife to go to the toilet when she gets
up in the morning, every couple of hours during the day, and
last thing at night. If she empties her bladder often there
may be fewer accidents. You may also notice signs that mean
she wants to go to the toilet. For example, she may fidget or
pace around. If this happens, prompt her to go to the toilet.
Ensure the toilet is easily accessible, warm and well lit.

Incontinence pads will soak up small volumes of urine and
can give you both confidence to leave the house. These come
in different varieties and it's worth speaking to a continence
adviser about them. Other things to consider include having
waterproof covers for your wife's usual chair, car seat and
mattress. Continence advisers will have various ideas that
may help you. Your GP should be able to put you in touch.

Incontinence can lead to sore skin, so your wife will need
bathing or showering at least daily. In between times, it may

be necessary to clean her with baby wipes. If your wife's skin does become red and sore, speak to her doctor as your wife may have a fungal infection that can be easily treated with the right cream.

Incontinence will mean a lot more work for you. Many people find it upsetting and distasteful. You may begin to feel angry and bitter. This is very understandable, but do try to talk to people about the problem and your feelings. Your GP, hospital specialist, district nurse, social worker and continence adviser will all have come across this before and will be able to help.

My mother has developed a habit of putting pieces of used toilet paper down the back of the bathroom radiator. When I ask her about this, she denies that she has done it. How should I handle this?

It seems that your mother has forgotten what to do with the toilet paper she has used. She may also have forgotten how to flush the toilet. It is unlikely to be useful to confront her with what she is doing. If possible, stand outside the bathroom door and when you think she is ready, go in and help her to flush her used paper down the toilet.

When we are out driving, getting my wife to the toilet can be quite a problem, especially as I can't just take her to the door and leave her. What is the best thing to do if she needs to use a public toilet?

Many carers face just this problem. The best thing to do is to use the disabled people's toilets, which are now available in most public buildings. You will find that these toilets are large enough for you to go in with your wife and assist her if that is necessary.

In some places, such as motorway service stations, the disabled toilets are kept locked. The key is usually available from the kiosk or from the information desk. RADAR (see Appendix 1) have a national disabled toilet scheme and you can obtain your own key from them. You do not have to be a wheelchair user to qualify.

Sometimes, the disabled toilet is inside the Ladies or Gents. If it is inside the Ladies, the only option is to be bold enough to go in there with your wife. You will find that most people will be understanding and discreet. If you are challenged, you have a good answer of course.

Food and drink

My wife has only a very small appetite and often refuses to eat anything at all. How can I persuade her? Is it usual for someone with Alzheimer's disease not to want to eat?

This is a common problem in the later stages of Alzheimer's disease. It is quite possible that your wife no longer understands about eating what is put in front of her. She may not feel hungry, perhaps because she takes very little exercise, or she may no longer recognise what it is to be hungry. It is also possible that she is having problems chewing or swallowing (see p. 60).

Try to make mealtimes part of a calm, relaxed routine. Encourage your wife to eat, and praise her when she succeeds. Suggest that she might find it easier to use a spoon instead of a knife and fork. Or give her finger food if she prefers this. Do not criticise her if she makes a mess (see also p. 59). If she has problems chewing and swallowing, it may be simplest to liquidise her food. If she is very forgetful, you may need to prompt her to take another mouthful, or to chew or swallow it.

However, the most important thing is that even if your wife does not want to eat, you should try to make sure that she drinks enough fluids — approximately eight cups of fluid a day is a rough guide. Plenty of fluid prevents constipation and dehydration.

My mother, who has had Alzheimer's disease for some years now, still has a good appetite but has lost a great deal of weight and is now very thin. Is this loss of weight due to her Alzheimer's disease? Do you think I should give her vitamin supplements?

It does seem that loss of weight may be a feature of Alzheimer's disease, although more research is needed into this. A recent research study compared a group of people with Alzheimer's disease with a group of people with other dementias and with a group of older people who did not have dementia. All the people in the study were in hospital and all were receiving adequate nutrition. Although the circumstances of the people in each of the three groups were similar, the people with Alzheimer's disease lost weight more rapidly than those in the other two groups.

It is sometimes helpful to give vitamin supplements to people in the later stages of dementia, but it would be best to speak to your mother's doctor first. He or she will be able to advise you on which supplements, if any, might be best for your mother.

My husband, who has Alzheimer's disease, sometimes forgets that he has just had a meal. He then complains about being hungry and and says I never give him anything to eat. What can I do?

It is quite common for people who are confused to forget they have just had a meal. An added problem may be that your husband no longer knows when he has had enough to eat – probably because the disease has affected a so-called satiety centre in the brain.

If your husband asks for another meal when he has just eaten, the best plan is to try to distract him with some other activity. If this fails, you could offer him a non-fattening snack, such as a piece of raw carrot or a stick of celery, to eat while he is waiting. With luck, he will then forget that he was wanting a meal.

Why does my wife, suffering from Alzheimer's disease, want to eat sweets and chocolates all the time?

The disease may have damaged what is sometimes called a satiety centre in the brain. The satiety centre's normal function is to let people know when they have had enough to eat. Some people with Alzheimer's disease do not know when to stop eating food in general. Others, like your wife, keep wanting to eat sweet things. It may be that your wife's disease has affected a particular part of the brain that normally helps people control their intake of sweet things. Alternatively, it may just be that your wife has always been extremely fond of sweets and chocolates, but used to be able to resist them.

I am caring for my elderly father, who has recently been diagnosed with Alzheimer's disease. He seems to be very prone to constipation. Can you advise?

You should try to ensure that your father eats a balanced diet containing plenty of dietary fibre. Foods that have a high fibre content include wholemeal bread and pasta, bran, cereals, pulses and dried fruits. One simple way of increasing the fibre content in the diet is to add bran to cereals, stewed fruit and puddings. Your father should also be encouraged to eat plenty of fresh fruit and vegetables, which will provide him with vitamins as well as fibre. Drinking plenty of fluids during the day will also help guard against constipation, as will taking plenty of exercise.

If your father is unwilling to eat the foods that would be good for him, and continues to suffer from constipation, then his doctor will probably be able to help. It is important to treat constipation in someone with Alzheimer's disease because constipation can cause agitation and aggravate confusion. The doctor may advise laxatives such as Regulan or Fybogel, which contain added fibre, or lactulose, which is a different sort of laxative that can also be very effective. Any of these laxatives (but not some of the others that are available over the counter) can be taken daily without harmful effect. In a small number of cases, it may be necessary for a district nurse to come and give regular enemas.

If my wife with Alzheimer's disease wants to eat baked beans out of the tin is there any wrong in it?

No, there is nothing wrong. Caring for someone with Alzheimer's disease requires people to be flexible about eating habits. Do make sure, however, that the tin has only just been opened, so that the beans are fresh. Also make sure, if your wife is feeding herself, that she does not cut herself on the opened tin.

My mother can no longer use a knife and fork properly and makes a dreadful mess. I find this very difficult to manage. Can you advise?

It is important for your mother's sense of independence and self-esteem that you should encourage her to continue to feed herself for as long as possible. However, both you and she will probably find this frustrating at times. Try always to be as flexible and tolerant as possible, and remember that your mother cannot help her bad table manners. She will probably cope best if you can make mealtimes as relaxed and unhurried as possible. It will also help her if you praise her for eating and enjoying her food, rather than getting upset about the mess.

Cleaning up afterwards will be easier if you use a plastic table cloth. If your mother can't cope with a table napkin, you could encourage her to wear an easily washable smock when she eats. Try tactfully to encourage her to use a spoon rather than a knife and fork, but make sure the food is cut up well for her. Finger food can sometimes be a good alternative. Don't worry if she picks up other food with her fingers. To reduce confusion, it is a good idea to serve only one portion of food at a time. If possible, remove salt, pepper and sauces from the table as soon as they have been used.

It may be worth asking if an occupational therapist can call to give you further advice. Aids that might possibly be helpful include non-slip mats, plates with suction pads, plate guards and cutlery with easy-grip handles.

Why has my partner, who suffers from dementia, suddenly become a vegetarian? He used to love meat.

A possible reason is that he no longer recognises meat for what it is, and that he finds it difficult to chew and swallow compared to some softer foods. (Also see the next answer.)

My wife, who has had Alzheimer's for some time now, finds chewing and swallowing a great problem. I find it very upsetting and I just don't know what to do.

Problems with chewing and swallowing do sometimes occur in the later stages of Alzheimer's disease and can be very upsetting. The most likely cause is that the muscles and reflexes involved in chewing and swallowing are no longer working so well. Sometimes, however, a person's chewing problems are due simply to ill-fitting dentures or sore gums, which can be sorted out. It might be useful to ask for professional advice.

The most important thing for you to try to accept is that your wife needs only a very small amount of food. This can easily be given in liquid form. A small amount of liquidised food, given at regular intervals, together with plenty to drink, will probably be quite adequate. If you can manage to be reasonably relaxed about all this, and can help your wife to take sufficient food for her needs, then you do not risk subjecting her to more undignified, uncomfortable and even hazardous methods of feeding.

My husband, who has Alzheimer's disease, was formerly a strict one-drink-before-supper man. Now he

makes too many visits to the drinks cupboard, with disastrous results. If I remove the bottles, he is still capable of going out to buy more. What should I do?

It seems that your husband has always liked to drink in moderation and it will probably be best for him if he is able to continue this habit. Obviously he should not be allowed to drink alcohol if he is taking any tablets that might react badly with it. Your husband's doctor or a pharmacist will be able to advise you on this.

The most likely reason for your husband's present drinking problem is that he forgets when he has already had a drink and so has another. You may need to be fairly imaginative in dealing with this, perhaps keeping the drinks cupboard full of bottles of water, limiting his money and encouraging people working in the local shop not to sell him alcohol. At the same time, it is reasonable to ensure that he can have a drink with his main meal each day. It might also be worth bearing in mind that he might be bored and might drink less if you could find him some distracting activities.

Taking pills

My mother has been prescribed a new drug for her Alzheimer's disease, but I know she'll forget to take it. What can I do?

Your mother has probably been prescribed one of the new anticholinesterase drugs (see p.156), such as donepezil or rivastigmine. Drugs of this type must be taken daily in order to have a chance of improving your mother's condition.

If someone can prompt her to take her tablets every day, even by a telephone call, then this could help. Another possibility is to get her to use a compartmentalised box, such as a Dosette or Medidose box. These boxes, which are available from chemists, have a different compartment for each day of the week. You, or another carer, could then help your mother by popping a tablet into a compartment for each day at the beginning of the week. Use of such a box might prompt your mother to take her medication. It will also provide her with an easy way of knowing whether or not she has already taken a tablet.

My husband is on a number of different tablets from the doctor. I am not sure what they are all for, but I have great difficulty getting him to swallow them all, especially the very large ones. What should I do?

It is quite common for people with dementia to be reluctant to take tablets. The problem usually occurs because people fail to recognise that there is anything wrong with them, and so do not appreciate the need to take medication. A problem with swallowing pills also sometimes occurs in the later stages of dementia as part of a more general difficulty with swallowing (see p. 60).

The first thing to do is to speak to your husband's doctor. The doctor will then be able to tell you what the various tablets are for, and also whether some tablets are more important than others. It might then be possible for you to concentrate your efforts on getting your husband to take just some of the tablets.

It is sometimes possible for a doctor to cut down on the total number of tablets that are being prescribed. Often, however, this will not be possible because the tablets are needed to treat a serious disorder, such as high blood pressure, heart failure, diabetes or epilepsy.

If your husband has a general problem with swallowing, it may be possible for him to have some types of medication in liquid form. Alternatively, it may be possible for some tablets to be crushed and mixed with food. A doctor or pharmacist will be able to advise you on this.

At some point it may be necessary for you to decide how far you are prepared to go to get your husband to take medication. Some carers feel very concerned about the ethics of tricking or forcing someone to take medication against their will. Others feel less concerned provided they are convinced that the medication is in the person's best interest. In almost every case, the use of physical force is likely to be counter-productive.

Sleeping

My wife, who has Alzheimer's disease, hardly seems to sleep and I am getting very tired as a result. I have been told that it is best to avoid giving her sleeping pills if possible, but what else can I try?

A range of practical measures can sometimes provide an effective alternative to sleeping pills. For example, you may be able to help your wife to sleep better if you can: provide plenty of activity during the day; stop her taking cat-naps; avoid giving her tea or coffee; keep the evenings fairly quiet; avoid giving her a heavy meal late at night; make sure the bedroom is warm and comfortable. (Also see the next answer for more information.)

If practical measures fail to improve matters, and if your own tiredness is making it difficult for you to cope, it may be necessary to reconsider giving sleeping pills. In general, these pills are best avoided when someone has Alzheimer's disease because of the risk of increased confusion. However, sometimes they can be the best solution. (See p. 158 for more information on sleeping pills.)

Some days my husband sleeps all day and then of course he is awake all night. As a result I get no sleep at all and become very irritable. What can I do?

Your husband is probably disorientated in time and does not recognise the difference between night and day. Try to establish a routine that will keep him as busy and active as possible during the daytime. (Information on activities is given in Chapter 5.) Unless you want to take advantage of a much needed break, don't let him take cat-naps. You may find that he sleeps better at night if you can keep him awake during the day. If he falls asleep in a chair during the day, gently wake him up.

To help him sleep at night, make sure that he is comfortable in bed and that the room is neither too hot nor too cold. Thick curtains to cut out the light will be helpful. If he will not settle easily in a bed, then he may sleep quite comfortably in a large chair or on a sofa.

Before he goes to bed at night, make sure that he uses the toilet. This will make him less likely to wake at night and will also help avoid possible bed-wetting. If he does get up during the night, try gently reminding him that it is still night-time. You might then be able to lead him quite easily back to bed. Another possibility is to distract him for a while and then suggest that it is time for you both to go to bed. Be as firm and reassuring as possible.

5
Communication and activities

Introduction

As Alzheimer's diseases progresses, communication becomes
more difficult. People with dementia develop problems both
in expressing themselves clearly and in understanding what
is being said to them. Communication problems can be
very frustrating and upsetting for everyone concerned – for
carers and sufferers alike. This chapter aims to help carers
to preserve the channels of communication for as long as

they possibly can. Also included in this chapter are practical suggestions for helping people with dementia to make the most of their failing memories. Finally, the chapter looks at ideas for keeping people with dementia occupied, so helping them to have as enjoyable a time as possible.

Improving communication

My mother's Alzheimer's disease is getting worse and I am desperate not to lose the ability to communicate with her. Can you advise me?

Communication does become increasingly difficult as Alzheimer's disease progresses. However, there are quite a number of things that you can do to help you and your mother to communicate:

- Make sure that she can see, hear and speak as well as possible (check hearing aids, glasses and dentures).
- Attract your mother's attention before you speak to her, perhaps by gently touching her arm.
- Try to avoid other distractions, such as from a television (tell her first that you would like to turn it off so that you can talk to her).
- While you are conversing with her, try to keep your head and shoulders at the same level as hers.
- Try to maintain eye contact when either of you is speaking (this will help keep her attention).
- Hold her hand during your conversation (another way of keeping her attention).
- Try to remain as calm as possible.
- Speak as clearly as you can.
- Use short sentences and try to talk about only one thing at a time.
- Give your mother plenty of time to answer or to show that she has understood.
- Write things down if your mother finds this helpful.

- Watch your mother's body language for visual clues as to how she might be feeling.
- Remember that you also can communicate non-verbally with your mother, for example by your facial expressions or by giving her a hug.

My husband, who has Alzheimer's disease, often starts to tell me something and then is unable to go on. It is so frustrating for both of us. What can we do?

It may help your husband if he knows that he has your full attention when he is speaking. You can convey this to him by maintaining eye contact throughout the conversation. He may also find it helpful if you gently nod your head from time to time to show that you are following what he is saying. If he loses track of what he is telling you, try to help him to continue by giving him a tactful prompt based on what he has already told you.

Remember that touch can often be a valuable aid to communication. Holding your husband's hand while he speaks will not only help him to maintain his concentration, it will also help to provide security in what must sometimes be for him a very baffling world. Such non-verbal communication is even more important in the later stages of Alzheimer's disease, when normal communication sometimes becomes impossible.

As communication with your husband becomes more difficult, it is very important for you to have your own opportunities for conversation. Friends, family members, neighbours, other carers, even the local shopkeeper can all help you with this.

My wife thinks she does all the chores, such as the cooking and shopping, and cannot accept that I now have to do everything. How can I explain this to her?

Your wife is no longer able to remember what she has just done. However, she can remember doing household chores on many previous occasions, and these are what she is remembering now. There really is no point in trying to explain the situation to her. She will not be able to acknowledge or thank you for all the extra work you are doing. It may help you to feel better if you can sometimes remind yourself that without your devotion and care it would not be possible for your wife to continue to live at home.

Memory aids

Does exercising the brain slow down the progress of dementia?

There is no clear answer to this question, but some research suggests that a person with dementia may possibly be helped by being gently encouraged to use his or her brain. Great care must be taken, however, not to overwhelm the person with mental exercises – such as reading, playing games, painting, etc – which could precipitate a crisis as the person realises that he or she is no longer capable of doing simple things. Provided that this is avoided, and the person with dementia continues to feel safe and secure, there is probably no harm and possibly some benefit in maintaining an environment that provides some stimulation.

My wife is in the very early stages of Alzheimer's disease and is frustrated by her loss of memory. What can I do to help her?

A useful way of helping your wife cope with her loss of memory is to encourage her to make the most of everyday memory aids and also to devise personalised 'memory joggers'. We all rely on information given by clocks, calendars, diaries, newspapers and so on. People with memory problems need these everyday aids all the more. They will also find it easier to manage if they can have their own memory joggers, such as message boards, handy lists and instruction sheets.

It will probably be most useful if you and your wife can work together to devise a range of memory aids to suit her particular needs. However, here are number of points and aids that you might like to consider:

- Keep familiar objects in their usual places, where your wife can easily see them.
- Make sure that watches and clocks show the correct time.
- Indicate today's date on any calendars, perhaps by marking off the days as they pass.
- Put up a message board in a prominent place and establish a habit of using it.
- Make a list of the day's activities and put it somewhere that it can be easily found. Encourage your wife to refer to it often and to tick off each activity as it is completed.
- If she has to be left alone while you go out, leave a clear note saying where you have gone and when you are due back. Try to establish a regular pattern so that your absences are part of a routine.
- Put up photographs of family members and close friends, all clearly named. Or add names to pictures in an album and encourage her to look at them often.

I get so frustrated because my wife forgets things that have just happened. Is it possible to re-train the memory of someone with Alzheimer's disease?

One of the main problems with Alzheimer's disease is the failure of short-term memory. This means that people forget things that have just happened. If you think about it, without looking at your watch, you could have a fairly good guess as to what time of day it is. You would also probably be able to remember when you last had a drink, what you had for breakfast and what month of the year it is. Such things tend to get lost in Alzheimer's disease, and people become confused as a result. For example, they may forget that they have just eaten lunch and ask for lunch again.

Most people think it is not possible to re-train the memory of someone with Alzheimer's disease. It may, however, be possible to help them to devise memory aids and joggers to help them function better, at least in the early stages of the illness. For example, a person with Alzheimer's disease might be able to continue to make a cup of tea if he or she has the instructions for doing this written down on a card. It would, however, still be necessary for the person to remember to look at the card and to be able to follow the steps one by one. Some people find message boards and scribble pads useful in the early stages of the illness. (Also see the previous answer for more memory-jogging ideas.)

My wife has Alzheimer's. Is it a good thing to keep going over the events of the day with her to try and help her remember them? Or is this a waste of time?

Even if you go over them with her, your wife will not be able to remember things which she has just done or which have just been said. This loss of short-term memory is one of the main symptoms of Alzheimer's disease. The best thing to do is to try and enjoy things together at the time of doing them. It is probably only upsetting for you and her if you keep reminding her of things that she cannot remember.

Activities

My husband is in the early stages of Alzheimer's disease. How can I keep him occupied?

In the earlier stages of the condition, it will not be too difficult to keep your husband occupied. He will probably be happy to help you with everyday household tasks, such as dusting and polishing, and laying and clearing the table. It does not really matter if he forgets what he has done and does these things again and again. He may also be able to help you with preparing food and doing the washing up. If you have a garden, this can present plenty of opportunities for simple activities.

A daily walk will probably do you both good and will also provide topics of conversation. If you keep an eye on him, he is likely to be able to go with you to the local shops. If he has been used to going to the pub or eating out, it is a good idea to help him to continue to do so for as long as he can. To avoid possible embarrassment it may be sensible to have a quiet word with the manager. It might also be a good idea for your husband to go to a day centre (see p. 72 and p. 116).

Assuming that he is fairly sociable, your husband will probably enjoy having friends and relatives to visit him at home. Generally, it is best to avoid large gatherings as these will be more difficult for him to cope with. If possible, warn any prospective visitors beforehand if they are not already aware of your husband's problems with his memory.

While your husband is still in the early stages of the illness, it would be a good idea to help him to prepare a scrapbook of his life, containing photographs and other souvenirs of earlier days. This will help him to remember his past for longer as the disease progresses. It could also be useful later on for strangers who may be helping to look after him. They will be able to go over the scrapbook with him.

Keeping your husband occupied in the later stages of the illness will be more of a problem, but it is worth making the effort. This will not only help him to get the most from life but will also help prevent other health problems – such as those that might arise from lack of exercise. Gentle exercises, such as moving to music, are often very popular. Repetitive tasks, perhaps based on previous interests, can be useful for maintaining interest and passing the time. Your husband may like being read to, and also listening to music – even if he wants the same piece over and over again!

My husband still enjoys going out on his own and finding his way home. However, he always goes to the

same shop – a local optician's. He stands at the counter and makes conversation. Eventually he leaves but he seems to have developed a fixation on this particular shop. What can I do about it?

This sounds to be a fairly harmless activity. It is probably best to explain to the shop assistant what your husband's problem is and suggest that they find ways of reassuring him and gently telling him to go back home. If you are worried about your husband getting lost, you might consider getting him to carry some form of identification (see p. 80).

My mother has been diagnosed with Alzheimer's disease but is still living on her own with her two cats. She is very attached to them. Do you think it will be all right for her to keep them?

Keeping animals may be beneficial to some people with Alzheimer's disease, especially in the early stage of the illness. Animals provide companionship and help keep people active. As long as you feel that you mother is able to care properly for her cats, then it would be best to leave them where they are. If you think she is not coping, then it would be best to make other arrangements. If you or one of your mother's neighbours could take the cats, then your mother would still be able to see them. If not, then discuss the problem with the local Cats Protection League or RSPCA.

Research has shown that contact with animals is helpful to elderly people living in residential homes.

It has been suggested that my wife should start going to a day centre. What sort of activities will there be at the centre for someone with Alzheimer's disease?

Day centres vary, but a variety of activities will probably take place. What exactly happens depends on how many people attend, how severe their dementia is and how well trained the staff are.

Practical help given at a day centre may include bathing, hairdressing and chiropody. Lunch is usually provided. Other activities, often done in groups, may include listening to music, doing simple exercises, and reminiscence therapy (see p. 166). Sometimes outings to shops and local places of interest may be organised. (Also see p. 116 for more information about day centres.)

Holidays

My husband and I always enjoyed our holidays together. He is probably getting too confused to go on an ordinary holiday but is there any way we could go together? I could really do with a holiday myself.

There are may kinds of holiday venues that cater for people with different disabilities and which will make you and your husband welcome. They range from private guest houses to well-equipped specialist holiday centres. If you choose the right one you will find that people are sympathetic and understanding of your difficulties.

RADAR publishes a directory of holidays for people with disabilities and also has information on access, insurance, other clients, outings and so on.

Some Alzheimer's Disease Society branches organise group holidays and many arrange day trips for people with dementia and their carers. The Alzheimer's Disease Society also has an arrangement with the Winged Fellowship Trust, a charity that provides holidays for people with disabilities. Special weeks are set aside in their special holiday centres for people with dementia and their carers. Contact the Winged Fellowship Trust to find out more.

Alzheimer Scotland has a holiday home at Cramond near Edinburgh. This is available for group bookings as well as for individual bookings at certain times of the year. In Scarborough and in Worthing, the Alzheimer's Disease

Society has a self-catering holiday flat for rent and it may be possible to arrange some care in the nearby day centre.

(See Appendix 1 for addresses of relevant organisations.)

I am planning a holiday with my mother who has Alzheimer's disease. Shall I need to mention her illness to the insurance company?

Yes, you must tell them or the insurance will not be valid. If your mother were to fall ill while on the holiday, the company might refuse to pay out.

Some companies might refuse to insure your mother altogether. Others will consider cases individually but may charge a higher rate. Advice on choosing an insurance company is available from RADAR (address in Appendix 1).

We have been planning a holiday for some time now to visit our son and his young family in Australia. However, my wife has just been diagnosed with Alzheimer's disease. Do you think we should still go?

As your wife has only recently been diagnosed, she may still be able to make this trip. A trip to see family members can be very important. However, it would be wise to seek advice from the doctor as your wife's ability to cope with the trip will depend on her particular condition.

People with even mild dementia may find long-haul travel especially difficult. In addition to the journey itself and subsequent jet-lag, your wife may be disorientated by the new environment.

If you do decide to go, you will need to take advice on travel insurance for your wife (see the previous question).

6

Personal safety

Introduction

Questions on topics relating to the personal safety of people with Alzheimer's disease become increasingly important as the dementia progresses. This chapter draws attention to a range of commonly met dangers, both inside and outside the home. It offers carers useful advice on how they might help to reduce the risk of accidents, while still allowing the people they care for to have as much independence as possible.

Living alone

My father shows signs of increasing confusion. How can I tell when it's no longer safe for him to live alone?

It is difficult to make a hard and fast rule. Many confused people do survive on their own for years in apparently hazardous conditions. They can even be helped to do so by a commonsense appraisal of the surroundings and the removal of the most obvious dangers.

There are, however, a number of key pointers to a person's inability to continue living alone. You should take account of these warning signs:

- carelessness with regard to unavoidable fire hazards (gas fires are the worst);
- leaving his home, particularly at night, and failing to find the way back;
- repeated complaints and expressions of anxiety by neighbours who were previously tolerant and helpful;
- a state of squalor that is inconsistent with the confused person's previous personality and personal dignity.

People have a right to live in their own home if at all possible and you should try to help your father to do so if he wants to (see Chapter 9 for information on getting help). The Alzheimer's Disease Society (see Appendix 1) has a useful booklet, 'Safe as Houses', with advice on how to reduce the risks for people with dementia who are living alone.

Dangers at home

My mother still prefers to live on her own even though she has dementia. I am particularly worried that she will have an accident with the gas. What can I do?

British Gas keeps a Gas Care Register of those customers who need special attention and special services. If your mother is not already on this register, you should telephone British Gas and ask for her to be included. It is also worth noting that free gas safety checks are available from British Gas to people living alone who are registered disabled, on Disability Benefit or over 60 years old. If the gas safety of your mother's home has not been checked recently, you should arrange a check as soon as possible. It will probably be useful if you can be present when the check is carried out. This will be reassuring for your mother and will give you the opportunity to ask questions if you need more information.

If your mother is in the habit of turning on gas taps without lighting the gas, it may be possible for British Gas to fit an isolation tap. A temporary solution might simply be to unplug your mother's gas cooker at the back. Obviously, she would then be dependent on someone else to do her cooking for her. If your mother is going to continue using gas, it might be useful to ask British Gas to fit a gas detector. However, such a device will only be of use if your mother is able to respond appropriately if it goes off.

My elderly aunt with dementia still lives alone, with morning and evening visits from home care-workers. Sometimes she forgets to turn the lights off and I'm worried she will leave an electric fire on and cause a fire. Is there anything I can do?

If the wiring and the various electrical appliances in your aunt's home are not new, you may wish to have them checked by a qualified electrician. Sometimes the Electricity Company will do this free of charge.

You might also advise her to use one of the safer forms of electric heating. For example, modern fan heaters and oil-filled electric radiators are both generally safer than radiant bar electric fires. Also, a circuit breaker between an electrical appliance and the electricity socket will provide added safety. If your aunt has central heating, it might be better to get rid of electric fires altogether.

Time switches would provide a simple means of ensuring that your aunt's lights and electrical appliances are turned on and off at appropriate times. The various switches could be set and checked by the home care assistant. It would also be a good idea to tell the electricity company of your aunt's special needs. Most electricity companies keep a register of older customers and those at possible risk.

My father, who has Alzheimer's disease and now lives with us, is a smoker. I worry about the possibility of fire. How can I stop him smoking?

The chances are that as your father's illness progresses he will forget about smoking. You may be able to bring this time forward if you remove his cigarettes and then don't do anything to remind him about smoking. If you smoke yourself, you should probably also stop or at least go and smoke somewhere that he cannot see you.

If your father becomes very agitated when you remove his cigarettes, it is probably wisest to let him continue smoking for a while before repeating your withdrawal tactic. You could meanwhile try to encourage him to cut down on the number of cigarettes he smokes and get him to try nicotine patches. For as long as he continues to smoke, you and other people who care for him will need to try to supervise him whenever he has a cigarette. Make sure his clothes and furniture are fire-resistant and that waste-paper bins are not near where he sits. A smoke alarm is always a good idea.

My wife, who suffers from Alzheimer's disease, has fallen several times in the house recently. Can you suggest how I might reduce the risk of falls?

Trying to make the home as hazard-free as possible makes good sense for everyone. It is particularly important when a person's risk of falling is increased by old age or confusion. Some common hazards that should be dealt with include:
- loose or torn carpet, especially on the stairs or in doorways;
- loose mats;
- highly polished floors;
- broken or loose stair rods;

- inadequate rails on the stairs;
- poor lighting (it would be worth having night lights if your wife often gets up at night);
- trailing electric flexes;
- wobbly or damaged furniture;
- furniture with protruding legs;
- clutter, such as shoes or newspapers, left on the floor;
- inadequate bathroom safety (see p. 51);
- worn slippers or other footwear that may cause tripping.

If you think you need further help, your wife's doctor or someone from Social Services will probably be able to arrange for an occupational therapist to come and advise you.

My husband has had a number of quite bad falls. So far our son has always been around to help, but I am 85 and would not be able to lift my husband on my own. What should I do if he falls when we are alone?

If your husband falls and is in pain, the best thing to do is to cover him with a blanket, give him a pillow if he can move his head freely, reassure him and tell him that you are going to get help. Then either telephone the doctor if the fall seems serious, or seek help from someone nearby.

If your husband appears to be unhurt, try putting a chair beside him and then encouraging him to use the chair to try to get up while you give him as much help as you can. If he can't understand what to do or if he is unable to get up when he tries, make him comfortable and then seek help.

Wandering

My father, who has Alzheimer's, still likes to go for short walks on his own. I am worried that he will get lost and come to harm. What precautions can I take?

If your father's walks take him out for only a short while,

and he is currently returning without much difficulty, there is probably not too much cause for concern. Indeed, the exercise he gets should be beneficial to both of you.

It would be sensible to make sure that your father always has his name, address and phone number on him. If you think that he would be happy wearing one, you may wish to purchase a special Medic-Alert bracelet or SOS talisman bearing the essential contact information. Alternatively, you could have a bracelet tag engraved at a local jewellers.

Another precaution would be to inform your local police station that your father has problems with his memory and his sense of time and place. Similarly, it is advisable to make sure that neighbours, the local shops and any other likely destinations are aware of the problem.

You should prepare yourself for the likely decline in your father's memory, which may cause him to get temporarily lost. It is very worrying when someone goes missing. If they do, alert the neighbours and also the police. It is unusual for anyone with Alzheimer's disease to go missing for 24 hours or more.

My wife, who has Alzheimer's disease, has been wandering out of the house and has once done this at night. My family keep telling me that I should ask the doctor for some medication. Can you advise?

It is best to avoid medication because the amount needed may produce undesirable side effects, such as drowsiness, falls and incontinence (see p. 158 for more about sleeping pills). It is better to make your home as secure as possible, ideally fitting bolts to the tops and bottoms of all outer doors.

My husband keeps wandering out of the house and getting lost. I feel so guilty when he keeps being brought back by the police. Why does he do this?

No one can be expected to keep a 24-hour watch on someone else so you should not blame yourself or others who have been left in charge of your husband. Wandering is quite common in people with dementia.

There are various possible reasons why your husband may be wandering. If he has always been an active person, it may simply be that he has excess energy which he needs to use up. Alternatively, he may be wandering to relieve boredom caused by poor concentration. A further possibility is that he may be looking for someone or something in his past which he just cannot remember.

My wife has wandered off and got lost several times. She has always come back home or been brought back, but I never know what to do. Can you advise?

Although it is very worrying when people with dementia get lost, they are not likely to come to any harm. The risk to your wife will obviously vary depending on where she gets lost.

As a general piece of advice, the best thing you can do if your wife goes missing is to try to remain calm and not panic. A first step might be to check the various places where your wife is known, such as your local shops. You should tell neighbours and friends.

It is generally best to contact the police sooner rather than later. To help the police and other searchers, it would be a good idea to keep a recent photograph of your wife close at hand and also to be able to give a clear description of the clothes she is wearing.

Driving

How can I persuade my husband, who has Alzheimer's disease, that he is no longer safe to drive a car?

Some people with Alzheimer's disease realise that they are no longer safe and give up driving easily. However, many others, like your husband, have no understanding that their skills are diminishing and that they no longer have the usual reactions or memory for driving. This can be an extremely difficult problem to manage.

If you don't need to use the car yourself, you should consider selling it so that your husband is not constantly reminded of it. If you want to continue driving the car, one possibility would be to make it difficult for your husband to find the car keys and then find ways of distracting him whenever he suggests driving. If you go out together in the car, you could suggest that you need the driving practice as you are a less experienced driver than he is.

Anyone affected by a medical condition that impairs their ability to drive is legally bound to inform the DVLA (see Appendix 1). If your husband is unable or unwilling to do this, you or his doctor should inform the DVLA on his behalf. The DVLA may offer a repeat driving test if necessary.

After your husband has stopped driving, you may be able to help him to retain his sense of independence if you suggest that he organises a taxi or mini-cab account.

Is it true that people with dementia can drive a car?

Research suggests that many people with dementia continue to drive after the onset of the illness, but in an unsafe fashion. However, a small number of people with dementia seem to preserve their driving ability. This is possibly associated with the fact that people in the early stages of dementia may still retain the ability to do things which they learned earlier on in their lives.

The main problem is that as dementia progresses, so the ability to drive inevitably deteriorates, but usually without the affected person realising that this is happening. It is very important that anyone who has become an unsafe driver should not be allowed to continue driving, however upsetting this may be.

7
Coping with difficult behaviour

Introduction

Alzheimer's disease and other dementias sometimes cause people to behave in ways that are difficult to manage. For example, people with dementia may become restless or aggressive for no obvious reason. It is important to remember that their behaviour is due to the illness and that they are not behaving badly on purpose. This chapter gives suggestions for managing some of the more common problems.

Being deliberately annoying?

Sometimes my wife does very silly things and then looks at me blankly. I get the feeling that she is being deliberately annoying. Can this be the case?

It is very unlikely that this is the case. Most people who have looked after someone with dementia have at some time or another felt that they are being taken for a ride or that the other person is being deliberately mischievous. People with dementia often do child-like things or may just appear bewildered or perplexed at times. This is a result of the illness. It is not a deliberate attempt to annoy.

As your wife's dementia advances, her difficult behaviour may make you feel increasingly bitter and angry. Don't feel guilty about these feelings. They are extremely common. If you discuss this with your local carers' group, you will be surprised how many other people feel the same way.

Repetitive questioning

My husband, who has Alzheimer's disease, keeps on asking me the same question over and over again. How can I learn to be patient?

This can be very irritating. The most likely cause is that your husband's memory problems are giving him a general feeling of insecurity. It may help you to be more patient if you can remember that it is very difficult for people with Alzheimer's disease to understand fully what is going on around them. You may also find the following ideas useful.

Sometimes, instead of answering the question for the umpteenth time, tell your husband that everything is fine and that you are taking care of things. Try to make him feel more secure. It might also help if you write the answer down. If he asks you the question again, you can then direct him to the written answer instead of answering the question yourself.

If your husband continues to ask one particular question, despite answers and reassurances, try to distract him by changing the subject or hugging him. Also, when he is not asking the question, give him lots of love and affection. Eventually (and it may be a while) he may stop asking it.

Losing things

My mother, who has dementia but still lives on her own, keeps losing her pension book. However, I always find it somewhere, usually under a cushion or under the bed but well out of sight. What can be done?

Your mother has dementia and it is inevitable that she will lose things. Eventually you might need to take charge of her pension book and other important documents yourself. In the meantime, you will probably discover her favourite hiding places. It would be wise to arrange for an Enduring Power of Attorney (see p. 134) if you have not already done so.

My father sometimes loses his keys and locks himself out of his flat. He wants to carry on living on his own although he has Alzheimer's disease. What can I do?

It would be a good idea to make several copies of your father's keys. You could then put one set in a safe place in your father's flat, keep one set yourself and ideally give a set to a helpful neighbour. Don't put your father's name and address on his keys in case a potential thief picks them up.

My mother frequently loses things and then accuses me and her home help of stealing them. How should we respond to, and deal with, these accusations?

Generally, you should try not to take these accusations too

seriously. Your mother's loss of memory increases the chance that she will misplace things. Because her things often go 'missing', she may well create her own safe hiding places for them. Unfortunately, she will also forget where these hiding places are, thus making the problem even worse.

It is usually pointless to contradict accusations of this type. You risk getting drawn into an argument with your mother, which may make her more upset. It is best to try searching for the object in question and to reassure her that you know where the missing item is. Try to discover any regular hiding places that she may have. Keep replacements of important items, such as spectacles and keys. Try to get into the habit of checking waste-bins before emptying them.

Try to make sure that your mother's home help, friends and neighbours understand the reason for your mother's behaviour so that they don't get upset.

It is worth bearing in mind that, occasionally, there may be some substance to accusations of theft made by people with dementia. If your mother's accusations involve purses or money in any form, you should always investigate as thoroughly as possible. Try to minimise her need to have cash or valuables in the house, so reducing any opportunity for theft by outsiders.

Depending on your mother's personality, you may have to prepare yourself for an increase in such accusations. Some people seem to be naturally more suspicious than others, and such personality traits may be exaggerated by dementia. Sometimes medication may help with this problem. Your GP will advise you as necessary.

Non-recognition

Sometimes, in the evenings, my husband looks at me and asks me when am I leaving. He then hands me the telephone and says 'Tell my wife to come home, so that you can go back to your home'. What can I do?

This can be a very distressing occurrence. This behaviour relates to your husband's poor memory and his inability to recognise you. He is remembering you as you were in the earlier part of his life. The best thing you can do is to give him a hug and remind him who you are. Then try to distract him, perhaps with a walk to the kitchen to make a cup of tea or some other activity which you can enjoy together.

My wife often says to me 'When are you going to take me home'. Then she packs some things into a bag – pictures, ornaments, etc. How can I explain that this is her home?

Home can mean so many things. It might mean the child-hood home that your wife may still remember as a place of safety, warmth and familiarity. People with dementia can find it difficult to relate to their surroundings. When they look around they may not recognise anything and this may make them feel very insecure or upset. You need to give your wife lots of hugs and reassurance. Tell her that this is her home, that all is well and that you are looking after her. It is best not to enter into any sort of argument with her. If she is convinced that she is not at home, you could try taking her out on a short walk with her bag and then return home and help her to unpack.

Hallucinations

My mother, who has Alzheimer's disease, seems to be having hallucinations. She holds conversations when there is no one there to talk to and seems to see things that don't exist. Sometimes she becomes very fright-ened and upset. How should I respond?

Hallucinations – in which people see, hear or sense the presence of someone or something that is not there – are quite a common symptom in Alzheimer's disease. It is not surprising that your mother sometimes becomes frightened and upset because hallucinations can seem very real.

If your mother becomes distressed by a hallucination, offer her reassurance and physical comfort by giving her a hug or holding her hand. Do not pretend that the content of her hallucination is real, but also do not get into any arguments about this. Keep as calm as possible and try gently to distract her, perhaps by offering her a drink or drawing her attention to something else in the room. Fortunately, even recurrent hallucinations usually last only a few days or weeks and then are forgotten.

Hallucinations are sometimes associated with poor vision, so it would be worth taking your mother to an optician to have her eyes checked. It will also probably help to keep rooms well lit as this will make your mother less likely to misinterpret what she is seeing. It would also be wise to talk to your mother's doctor. Medical treatment is sometimes helpful (see p. 162), or it may be necessary to adjust other medications that can cause hallucinations as a side effect.

Restlessness and agitation

My husband, who has Alzheimer's disease, gets sudden bouts of restlessness and I feel at my wits' end how to cope. Why is this and how should I manage?

Restlessness is a very common feature of Alzheimer's disease. It can make the affected person very agitated, and sometimes leads to wandering (see p. 79). Restlessness has a number of possible causes, some of which can be avoided.

If restlessness comes on suddenly, then it may be due to pain or discomfort. Toothache is a common cause of pain, which should always be investigated and treated. Digestive problems, such as indigestion and constipation, also commonly cause pain or discomfort, but can often be avoided if attention is paid to the diet (see p. 58). Discomfort due to a full bladder is an extremely common cause of restlessness, so it is worth ensuring that your husband visits the toilet frequently. If he has difficulty passing urine, he may have a urinary tract infection that needs medical attention.

Almost any drug your husband is on could cause restlessness. You should therefore check with his doctor to see if any of his medications might be reduced or stopped. Caffeinated drinks, such as tea or coffee, can also cause or aggravate restlessness and agitation.

Another possibility is that your husband's restlessness is due to boredom, in which case it might help if you can find more activities for him (see Chapter 5 for ideas). Sudden bouts of restlessness can often be relieved by going out for a walk or taking some other form of exercise.

If none of these suggestions works, it might mean that your your husband is feeling anxious and upset. In which case, it might help him if you give him hugs or sit with him for a while, perhaps holding his hand or reading to him.

I live with and look after my older sister, who has been diagnosed with Alzheimer's disease. She often becomes very agitated, especially in the afternoons. The doctor has not been able to find any particular cause for this. He does not think drugs would help her. What can I do to calm my sister down?

Although agitation may have a whole range of causes (including those given in the previous answer as causes of restlessness), it does sometimes occur as an inexplicable part of the disease itself.

You may be able to quieten your sister if you can respond calmly and gently to her agitation – although you may find this very wearing. It may sometimes help if she is given something simple but useful to do, such as posting a letter with you. Certainly you should avoid any complicated activities when she is already agitated. Often, with time, agitation gives way to a mood of emptiness and passive acceptance.

My elderly mother, who has dementia and lives with us, sometimes has screaming fits. Why is this and what can I do about it?

People with dementia often have a phase of screaming fits. The first thing you should do is to ask your mother's doctor to check for any possible physical reason for the screaming, such as pain or constipation. It may help the doctor if you notice whether there is any pattern to the screaming, for example is it just around mealtimes?

If no physical cause is found, it is probable that your mother just feels bewildered. Try to keep calm, hold her often and make her feel loved and supported. If the screaming persists, she may need a small amount of sedation from the doctor, as well as plenty of comfort from you. Usually this distressing phase passes and the sedation can be stopped.

I have noticed that my husband becomes much more disturbed towards the end of the day, just when I am feeling very tired. What can I do to calm him down?

The best advice is to try to keep the evenings fairly quiet. Encourage visitors to come early in the day if possible, when they may be less tiring or less likely to upset your husband. If you usually give your husband a bath in the evening, try changing this to the morning. It is possible that your husband realises when you are tired and that this affects how he behaves. If possible, try to find ways in which you could get some rest yourself earlier in the day.

Anger and aggression

When I try to explain to my wife that she has done or said something wrong, she becomes very defensive and angry and blames me and tells me to leave. I find this very upsetting. What can I do?

It is not surprising that you find this upsetting. However, you must remind yourself that your wife's problems are due to the disease. She cannot help it when she does or says something wrong. Having made the mistake, she may either want to conceal it, or have no recollection at all of what she has done. In either case, it would be best for you to try to avoid drawing attention to your wife's failures and to keep as calm as you can. Any type of conflict will be likely to cause distress both for you and your wife.

Sometimes I think my father must really hate me. He has Alzheimer's disease and I have moved in with him. I want to carry on caring for him but he gets so angry with me and says such awful things. What might I be doing wrong?

Although is natural for you to blame yourself, it is very important for you to understand that your father's anger is not really aimed at you. You are not causing his anger. The anger is part of his illness. It is common for people who have Alzheimer's disease to pass through a phase of being angry and sometimes aggressive.

Although this angry phase will pass, it may help you in the meantime to consider some of the things that may be triggering your father's anger. A community psychiatric nurse (see p. 115) could visit your home to help you with this.

There are many possible reasons why your father may be feeling so angry. For example, he may not like being forced to accept help to do things that he used to do on his own, such as washing. Or perhaps he feels frustrated simply because he is unable to do certain things. Another possibility is that your father is bewildered and frightened because he no longer understands what is going on around him. It is also possible that he is just bored or has an excess of energy. Sometimes, hunger, the need to pass urine, or constipation can lead to disruptive behaviour. If the angry outbursts have only started recently, they may be due to an infection or pain. Once you have been able to identify some of the things that tend to make your father angry, you may be able to reduce the number of angry outbursts.

My husband, who has Alzheimer's disease, often gets angry and sometimes hits me. He never used to do this. What can I do to calm things down?

It is important to remember that your husband's anger is not aimed directly at you – it is part of his disease (see the previous answer). You may find that you get very angry yourself and even want to hit him back. However, this is quite likely to make the situation worse. When this happens, try to react calmly. If you can manage to distract him he will probably quite quickly forget why he has been so angry. If you feel you are in any danger, it would be wise to leave the room for a while. You may also want to call a friend or neighbour.

Under certain circumstances, antipsychotic drugs, such as risperidone, may help to calm your husband down. You should talk to your doctor about the benefits and drawbacks of drugs of this type (see also p. 162).

Above all, try not to get disheartened or frustrated with the care you are giving your husband. This distressing phase always passes after a time. When your husband is calm give him plenty of love and affection.

My mother has dementia. She never used to swear but now she seems to swear all the time. It doesn't matter who is present. What should I do?

You are probably surprised that your mother even knows the words that she uses. The fact is most of us know these words, but would not usually bring them into our conversation. The normal brain has an inbuilt mechanism which tells us the difference between appropriate and inappropriate behaviour and language. When certain areas of the brain are affected by dementia or another disease, this mechanism is impaired. Swearing may be the only way in which your mother can express anger, anxiety, pain or discomfort.

You may find it useful to ask a community psychiatric nurse (see p. 115) or other health professional to help you to find out whether there are any particular situations that appear to trigger off your mother's bad language. You might then be able to help her to avoid these situations.

Sexual behaviour

Is it common for people with dementia to show unusual sexual behaviour?

People with dementia, both men and women, do sometimes display inappropriate sexual behaviour, although this is not common. Such behaviour may include undressing in public, fondling the genitals, or touching someone in an inappropriate way. The best way to respond is to try not to over-react and to remember that the behaviour is due to the disease. Then calmly and quietly try to distract the person and encourage some other activity.

My husband, who has Alzheimer's disease, wants to have sex with me much more than he used to. I can't cope with his excessive demands for sex and am finding it all very distressing. Sometimes I want to react by sleeping in a separate bed. What should I do?

It is very understandable that you feel upset. You may feel better if you are able to remember that your husband's changed sexual behaviour is part of his illness. Your husband probably does not remember that he has just had sex with you and this is why he wants to start again.

If your husband gets angry when you refuse him, you will probably find it best to keep out of his way until the moment has passed for him or he goes to sleep. This might mean going to sleep in a separate bed sometimes. Whether or not you want to sleep separately on a permanent basis is a more difficult decision. You will probably find it helpful to talk to someone who has been trained to help people to cope with sexual problems. People who might be able to help are your community psychiatric nurse, a counsellor specialising in sexual problems, or Relate (address in Appendix 1).

Other people's attitudes

We live in a flat and my husband, who has dementia, sometimes gets noisy and disturbing especially at night. I feel so embarrassed and ashamed. What should I tell our neighbours?

It might take some courage, but you will find it easier to manage in the long run if you apologise to your neighbours but also tell them that your husband has dementia and that he cannot help sometimes making a noise. If your neighbours have never heard of dementia, you may need to explain that it is a physical disorder of the brain that affects a person's memory, language and understanding.

My father, who has dementia, now lives with us and I am pleased to be able to care for him. However, my nine-year-old son no longer brings his friends home because he is embarrassed by his grandfather's behaviour. I am very sad about this. What can I do?

You should talk to your son about this. He may find it helpful to read the book 'It's Me Grandma! It's Me', published by the Alzheimer's Disease Society (See Appendix 1 for the address. The Society also produces a leaflet for teenagers on this subject.) Encourage your son to tell his friends about his grandfather's illness. With your support, your son might be able to bring his friends home, introduce them to his grandfather and then perhaps go off to his room to play.

8
Carers' emotions

Introduction

Caring for someone else can be a heavy burden. You may
have physical and health problems of your own. You may be
tired from lack of sleep or from the constant need to pay
attention to someone else. You may have worries from
financial problems or about how long you can cope. You may
just want a break. Your needs are just as important as the
needs of the person you care for. You have a right to health

95

and rest, to time for yourself, and to stop caring if you want to. You will be able to care better for someone else if you also care for yourself.

Emotional support

Since my wife became ill most of our friends have stopped visiting. How can we persuade people that Alzheimer's disease is not catching and that my wife and I need friends and visitors?

It's an old cliché that in times of trouble you find out who your real friends are. But your friends probably haven't stopped liking or caring for you. It's just that they don't know how to react to the change in your lives.

Try speaking directly to the people who have been closest to your wife and yourself. Phone them or go round to see them and explain about the illness. Let them know that you haven't changed and that you and your wife need company even more. If they are real friends then they will support both you and your wife.

As a carer you certainly need all the friends you can get. Try to get breaks from caring to keep up with your old social life – going to the pub, playing golf, going to the pictures, whatever you used to enjoy doing. You need to keep space and time for your own interests and activities.

Many carers find that they make new friends if they join a carers' support group or Alzheimer's Disease Society branch. Certainly there will be people there who understand your need for company. In some places there are visiting schemes where a volunteer will come and visit you and your wife on a regular basis.

Sometimes I feel so alone. As though there is only me and my husband in the whole world. He has dementia.

I don't need help. I just need someone to talk to. What can I do?

Having someone to talk to can be a great help for carers. Many people find that it is much easier to cope if they are able to share their feelings and experiences.

There are a number of different ways that you can contact people who will listen and understand. The Alzheimer's Disease Society and Alzheimer Scotland both have telephone helplines (see Appendix 1). The Alzheimer's Disease Society also has local carers' contacts who are trained volunteers willing to talk and assist you.

In some areas there are befriending schemes that will arrange for someone to visit you in your own home. If you want to get out of the house, then you will probably be able to find a carers' group that meets regularly somewhere not far from where you live. Such groups have been set up by many voluntary organisations and also by Social Services.

I'm a gay man and I care for my partner of twenty years who has dementia. I go to a carers' group but I don't feel very welcome. It's not that they are unkind but I know they don't think my relationship is the same as theirs or my pain as real. Is there anywhere I can get help from people who really understand?

Some carers' groups are better then others at making people welcome. It's a pity that the one you went to didn't help you as your experience of caring is the same as anyone else's and your feelings are just as important.

Many cities now have groups for gay carers. Most of them focus on caring for people with AIDS, some of whom develop dementia. You may find that one of these groups is relevant to your needs. Ring your local gay helpline to find out about carers' groups in your area, or contact the Terrence Higgins Trust (see Appendix 1).

The national Alzheimer's Disease Society (see Appendix 1) may be able to put you in touch with another gay carer.

Loss and despair

Sometimes I feel such a terrible sense of loss and despair now that my husband has Alzheimer's disease. It makes me just want to sit down and give up. How can I get help for my feelings?

You first started to help yourself when you admitted how overwhelming these feelings are. As Alzheimer's disease progresses, the illness robs us of the person we used to know. You may feel a great loss of companionship. In many ways it is like grieving for the death of someone who is still alive.

Grief is common among people like you who are caring for someone with a long-term illness. You may find yourself shifting between hope and despair, thinking your husband may get better and then knowing that he won't.

Don't be afraid of these feelings. They are real and natural. Try to focus on the small things you can do to make life as pleasant as possible for your husband, and look for the parts of his personality which are still there.

It always helps to find someone to talk to. Share your feelings with family and friends, join a carers' group or talk to your social worker, community psychiatric nurse or an Alzheimer's Disease Society carers' contact.

My father has had Alzheimer's for six years. He is very restless and nearly always distressed. He searches the house endlessly looking for my mother who has been dead for four years. He cries a lot. I just cannot find a way of comforting him. At night when he's asleep I think I could just smother him with the pillow and it would be better for both of us. I know that's not true but I'm scared I might do it. What can I do?

Such feelings are not uncommon. Dementia brings a terrible sense of loss to all of those involved. You feel a deep loss for your father as a person who once cared for you, he feels his whole life slipping away from him and longs for the security of the past as represented by his wife. It's very painful to see the distress of another person and be unable to help.

You must talk to someone about your feelings, perhaps a close member of the family, a friend, or the Alzheimer's Disease Society or Alzheimer Scotland helpline (see Appendix 1). Your feelings and your fears are nothing to be ashamed of. Try to get more breaks from caring. Talk to your doctor or social worker about how you can reduce your father's anxiety. Make sure they know how hard you are finding things and insist on having proper support and respite breaks (see p. 117). You should not have to take on this burden alone.

Anger and bitterness

Is it normal to get angry and lose my temper when my mother repeats things endlessly. Are all carers supposed to be saints?

No, you do not have to be a saint. Neither are other carers. You are an ordinary person doing your best at a very difficult task. Repetitive behaviour – such as endlessly asking the same questions, shouting or hiding things – is common among people with dementia and can be intensely irritating. It is not surprising that you sometimes lose your temper and feel that only a saint could go on.

Losing your temper probably isn't good for you and it certainly doesn't help your mother. Try to understand your mother's behaviour and see if you can stop it or reduce it (see Chapter 7 for suggestions). If you do feel you are going to lose your temper, try to go into another room or into the garden. Perhaps you will be able to scream or cry there, or just take a deep breath and calm down.

You don't have to manage these problems alone. Both the Alzheimer's Disease Society and Alzheimer Scotland have helplines (see Appendix 1). Many local Alzheimer's Disease Society groups have carers' contacts whom you can telephone and talk to. Best of all try to get advice from your doctor or from the local community psychiatric nurse (see p. 115) on ways of dealing with your mother's repetitive behaviour. Also make sure you ask for regular respite breaks (see p. 117).

My husband keeps wandering off and being brought back by the police. I get so angry and often end up shouting at him. I know this is not good for either of us. What should I do?

It is very natural to get angry in these circumstances. Anger is a common reaction after worry. You probably get angry at your husband because you have been very worried about him, fearing that something dreadful might have happened. You just have to tell yourself that your husband can't help it. Wandering is very common in people with dementia (also see p. 79). Whenever your husband is brought back home, he is likely to be very confused and frightened. Rather than being angry with him, you should try very hard to reassure him and comfort him and get him back into his familiar routine.

My husband follows me from room to room and even when I go to the toilet he stands outside the door. I feel I never have any space for myself, and this makes me very tense and prone to lose my temper at him. What can I do?

Your husband is following you around because he feels insecure. He probably thinks you are not going to return and that makes him feel very unhappy.

Whenever you leave the room, it is important to try to reassure your husband that you will be coming back in a few minutes. However, to get more space and time for yourself, it would be a good idea to ask a friend or a neighbour to sit with your husband sometimes. This will probably help you to feel more relaxed and may make it easier to cope with your husband's clinging behaviour when you return.

I don't mind looking after my mother, who has Alzheimer's and can't manage on her own, but I feel very bitter about my brother and his wife. They won't have her to stay and never come to visit. I've given up my job so we are on one income but my brother doesn't contribute anything financially. I think he last rang three months ago. What can I do about this?

Alzheimer's disease doesn't just affect the person who is ill, it affects the whole family and many different relationships. Sometimes one member of the family, like you, shoulders the whole burden, while others, like your brother, keep away and pretend the problems are not their responsibility. This often leads to bitterness and family feuds.

If you can possibly manage to talk to your brother, you should do so. Ask him to visit and try to make him face up to sharing the responsibility. It may be he is just scared of doing so, that he feels you are so much more caring than he is, or that he cannot accept your mother's illness.

If you cannot find a way for your brother to be involved, it would be better to look actively for help from elsewhere. Make sure you have all the breaks and respite care (p. 117) you need. Ask your social worker to help with any benefits you can claim (also see p. 138). If you really look after yourself, you may feel less stressed and less bitter about your brother.

Sexual feelings

My husband who has Alzheimer's disease seems to have lost all interest in having a sexual relationship with me. I am missing this aspect of my life and feel very guilty about feeling this way. What can I do?

It is very natural for you to feel this way. Everyone has a life-long need to be loved and touched, and sexuality is a normal part of adult life. Gentle cuddling and holding may be mutually satisfying, and will let you know if your husband is able or inclined to engage in further intimacy. Patience may pay off. Your husband's condition may vary from time to time and there may be days when he is more sexually inclined than others.

In this situation, some people find other sexual outlets, for example masturbation or an extramarital relationship.

Guilt

My wife has had Alzheimer's disease for eight years and I am feeling worn out in spite of a great deal of support. I know I should consider putting her in a home but I do not know how I am going to cope with the guilt of giving up caring. Can you advise me?

You have cared for your wife already for a very long time. Also, you have loved her and know her better than anyone else does. I am sure you always felt you would be able to continue to care for her indefinitely. Unfortunately, caring for someone with Alzheimer's disease becomes a 24-hour occupation and it is not normal for anyone to continue to care on this basis without any relief. I expect you have already had help from health services and Social Services and from your local Alzheimer's Disease Society group. However, there comes a time when short breaks of respite care just do not provide sufficient relief.

You should try to visit some homes and then introduce your wife to one of them gradually, getting her to stay there for short periods of time. Many homes are prepared to do this. In that way, the staff get to know her. If she goes there permanently, it should be possible for you to continue to care for your wife by helping at mealtimes and washing her. You can distract her and take her out and continue to contribute a great deal to her life. At the same time, you will be giving the staff of the home a great deal of support. Homes are very often under-staffed and, if you discuss with the home how best you can help them, this might go a long way towards relieving the guilt you feel. After all, I am sure you feel that your wife would not have wanted you to risk your own health by looking after her.

Since I put my mother in a nursing home I have felt such guilt. She was impossible to look after at home and we have two young children. But I can't get her distress over the move out of my mind. Have I done the wrong thing?

The decision to move someone they love into a care home is often one of the most difficult and painful decisions that carers ever have to make.

You have many responsibilities, to your children and to your husband as well as to your mother. Sometimes it is not possible for people to balance their various responsibilities, and hard decisions have to be taken. Sometimes your own needs have to come first. Sometimes the needs of the person you love are so complex that you cannot provide good care for them at home.

Feeling guilty won't help you or your mother. Face up to the decision and think about the advantages for you, your mother and your family. Try to concentrate on the positive care your mother is getting at the care home. Visit her as much as possible and encourage other members of the family and her friends to visit her too. Make sure she knows you haven't forgotten her and that you and the family still love her. Take your children with you if you can.

9

Getting help

Introduction

Getting the help that is needed when someone has Alzheimer's disease or another dementia is not always easy. There is a wide range of information and advice, services and support, but finding your way through to the different organisations and agencies which provide it can be difficult. The three key contacts are the GP of the person with dementia, the local Social Services department and the Alzheimer's

Disease Society. This chapter answers common questions about types of help and how to get it.

Sources of help and information

Where can I turn for help and information?

You are not alone. Many people and organisations, both professional and voluntary, can help make your caring task easier. Don't be afraid to ask. You will find a list of useful addresses and telephone numbers in Appendix 1, including those of the organisations mentioned below.

The Alzheimer's Disease Society has a national information service and many local groups. Your local branch will know about local services. It will also have as members many fellow carers, who will understand your worries and problems and be able to help you. If you join the Society you will receive a useful monthly Newsletter full of news and practical advice.

The Carers National Association is a support organisation for carers of all kinds. Age Concern will also help you. Expert advice on benefits and financial matters can be obtained from Citizens Advice Bureaux (CABx).

Your local Social Services department, if asked, will carry out separate assessments of both you (see p. 109) and the person you are caring for (see p. 108). His or her GP and hospital specialist will advise you on health services.

Are there training courses for people caring for someone with dementia?

There are many opportunities for family carers to learn about dementia and how to care for someone who has it. Branches of the Alzheimer's Disease Society (see Appendix 1) and local carers' groups often have speakers and may run practical sessions on topics such as difficult behaviour, safety aspects or lifting people. In some areas, more formal courses

are run by Social Services to help carers with their task.
There are also many conferences for carers organised at
regional and national level. You can find out about these
from the Alzheimer's Disease Society Newsletter or from
Alzheimer Scotland (see Appendix 1).

As part of its Care Learning Programme the Alzheimer's
Disease Society publishes the Carers Resource Pack, which
has the structure of a course and provides exercises for you
to do to confirm that you have learned what you have read.
There is a special version of the pack for carers of younger
people with dementia.

The Alzheimer's Disease Society has also produced a video
training course for carers, entitled 'Love is Not Enough'. This
video is intended for use by a group with a leader.

Spiritual needs

**My husband and I have always gone to our church on
Sundays. Although he doesn't understand much now,
he still seems to enjoy the services and to benefit from
them. I worry about other people, though, as he makes
disturbing noises. How can we try to meet the spiritual
needs of people with dementia?**

If you have a religious faith, then you will believe that a person with dementia retains their spiritual dimension intact
despite the disease. It is right, therefore, to try to meet those
spiritual needs. The ritual of familiar religious services can
be very helpful and calming for a person with dementia, and
people should be given the opportunity to attend their place
of worship for as long as they are able. The minister and
other worshippers will probably be very tolerant and helpful
if you explain the situation to them.

When someone with dementia is no longer able to go out,
a minister will visit them at home and say prayers or give
the sacraments as appropriate.

The Christian Council on Ageing (see Appendix 1) is concerned with the spiritual needs of people with dementia. Jewish Care (see Appendix 1) may also be able to help.

Community care

What is 'community care' and how do I get it?

Community care is a general term for services provided to help people with illness or disability to continue to live in their own homes. The policy of community care also encourages local provision of sheltered housing and of residential and nursing homes within the 'community'.

The arrangements for community care are set out in the Community Care Act (1992). The Act confirms Social Services departments' responsibility to assess people's needs (by a procedure known as a needs assessment, see p. 108) and to provide or purchase a range of services to meet those needs. There is a strong assumption that services will be provided to keep people in their own homes for as long as possible.

Community care has resulted in a growing number of different services designed to support people in their own homes (see p. 113). However, the range and level of services varies a great deal from area to area. Financial restraints sometimes mean that it is not possible for someone to be supported at home. Local authorities are not legally obliged to provide community care for individuals if this would cost more than moving them to a residential or nursing home, although they sometimes will

To obtain services provided by the NHS – such as nursing help or physiotherapy – you should ask the GP or hospital specialist of the person who is ill. To obtain other services – such as home helps or meals on wheels – first ask your Social Services department for a needs assessment under the Community Care Act. Then ask Social Services what they should and can provide to meet those needs. You can find out who to speak to by ringing the local Council offices. (See p. 113 for information about services that might be available.)

What is a 'needs assessment' for community care?

A needs assessment is organised by Social Services when they think that someone may need community care. The assessment will usually be carried out by a social worker or an occupational therapist. They will take account of the views of the person's GP and community psychiatric nurse (see p. 115) if there is one. As a carer or close relative, you should also be able to be involved and to contribute, since you probably know the person being assessed better than anyone else does. However, it is that person's assessment, not yours, and you must not mind if you are not included in every part of it. (You can also request your own needs assessment, see p. 109.)

The needs assessment will include reports from the various professionals who have been involved. It will also include a questionnaire. You need to be sure that the questionnaire is properly filled in. People who have Alzheimer's disease may not be able to answer the questions properly and you may need to do it for them.

After a needs assessment has been carried out, Social Services should discuss with you what services are available in your area to meet those needs. They should also appoint a care manager (see the next answer) to draw up and monitor a care plan for the person who has been assessed.

What is a care manager?

A care manager is a person, usually a social worker, who draws up and manages a care plan for someone who has had a needs assessment (see the previous answer). The care plan sets out the types of community care that should be available to meet the needs of the person who has been assessed.

The care manager is an important person for a carer to work with in the provision of care for a person who has

Alzheimer's disease. A good care manager will be very sup-
portive and a useful source of information and advice.

The care manager should provide you as a carer with a
copy of the needs assessment and also of the care plan, and
be prepared to discuss them with you. He or she should
monitor the care plan and make appropriate changes to it to
meet changing needs as the disease progresses. If you do not
see the care manager on a regular basis, you should contact
him or her whenever you feel that the needs of the person
you care for have changed or if you need extra help.

**What can I do if I don't agree with the needs assess-
ment or with the amount of help offered for my father
who has dementia?**

If you do not agree with the needs assessment or with the
care plan for your father, you should discuss the problem
with his care manager. If you cannot reach an agreement
with your father's care manager, you should follow the
complaints procedure which will be published by your Social
Services department.

**What about me? Care in the community is all very
well, but I seem to be doing most of the work looking
after my mother who has Alzheimer's disease.
Shouldn't my needs be considered as well as hers?**

If you are the main carer, and if you either share the
house with your mother or look after her on a regular and
substantial basis, then you can request your own needs
assessment. A carers' needs assessment is not a test of how
well you are caring. It is a way of checking if you are getting
the support you need to carry on caring if you want to.

Carers' needs assessments are carried out by Social
Services under the arrangements in the Carers (Recognition
& Services) Act (1995). A carers' needs assessment can be
considered only in conjunction with a needs assessment for
the person who is being cared for. If your mother has not

already had her own needs assessment, or if circumstances have changed, you will have to ask for her to be assessed as well. A social worker will visit you and your mother to talk about the help you need. You can ask to be assessed separately or together.

Unfortunately, having assessed your needs, Social Services are not under any legal obligation to provide you with help. However, if you are not offered any help, a carers' needs assessment will enable you to argue for more support or for respite care (see p. 117) if you want it. Remember Social Services are responsible for your mother, not you. Any support you give her is up to you so they must take account of her needs without taking your care for granted.

The Carers National Association (see Appendix 1) has a helpline that will provide advice on carers' needs assessments. This association also publishes an excellent booklet called 'New Rights for Carers'.

My mother has Alzheimer's disease but her GP isn't very helpful. The GP says my mother should go into a nursing home. My father wants my mother to stay at home with him. If this is to happen he needs a lot more help. What can I do?

The first step is for you to think very carefully about whether your father is likely to be able to cope with looking after your mother, and for how long. You also need to think about how much extra help might be needed to enable him to do this.

The GP's opinion is important but it is really for your family to decide together with Social Services what is best. The GP may know a lot about your mother's health but cannot decide where she should be cared for. You should ask Social Services for an assessment (or reassessment) of your mother's needs (see p. 108) and for a separate assessment for your father as a carer (see p. 109).

If a decision is made to keep your mother at home, and her GP is still unhappy about this, you may want to find her a more understanding GP. Even so, you should probably start thinking ahead to a time when your mother may be better off in a nursing home (see Chapter 10).

A few years ago I had a slight stroke. It has left me very weak on one side and a bit wobbly. Now my wife is getting confused. The doctor says its Alzheimer's disease. We want to go on caring for each other but I'm scared of the future. How can I care if I'm disabled?

If you have not already done so, ask Social Services to conduct a needs assessment (see p. 108) under the Community Care Act. They should also carry out a separate assessment of your needs (see p. 109). Make sure also that you are getting all the state benefits, such as Attendance Allowance, that you are entitled to (see p. 138).

The fact that your stroke has left you with strength and mobility problems will make some things more difficult for you, and where you live will make a lot of difference. You might want to consider moving into sheltered housing (see the next answer).

Try to make a realistic assessment of what you can and can't do and remember that your wife will need a lot more care later in her illness. With extra help, you and she may be able to continue caring for each other for a time. However, this may not be possible indefinitely, because her needs and perhaps also yours may become too great. Taking time now to plan for the future, such as investigating a possible move either into sheltered housing or a care home (see p. 122), is itself an important aspect of caring for someone.

I want to carry on looking after my husband who has dementia but my arthritis is making me less mobile than I used to be. Might a move into sheltered housing make things easier?

This type of accommodation is designed specially for people with mobility and care needs. Residents continue to live as independently as possible, in self-contained flats or in a complex of houses. The units may have fittings, such as easy-to-use taps and safety rails, to help people with mobility problems. They also have alarms for calling a warden in case of emergency. There will also probably be Social Services help with shopping, cooking and so on. There are some places now which are able to give more help as people's needs increase.

My next door neighbour, who lives alone, is getting more and more confused. I try to keep an eye on him but I'm worried about the safety in his home. What if he leaves the gas on? He doesn't seem to have any relatives. Who should I contact?

If Social Services are already helping your neighbour, for example if he has a home help or receives meals on wheels, you should share your safety fears with them.

If your neighbour is not already being helped by Social Services, the best thing to do is to let his GP know about your worries. GPs have to offer an annual health check to people over 75 and this may be a chance to get a reluctant person to see a doctor. The GP can then arrange for Social Services to carry out a needs assessment under the Community Care Act (see p. 108). If you can't find out the name of your neighbour's GP, then the best way of getting help for him would be for you to contact Social Services (address in the Phone Book).

On the specific question of gas safety, British Gas keep a Gas Care Register of customers who need special attention and special services. If it is not possible to ensure the safety of your neighbour, it may be necessary for Social Services to disconnect the cooker and to arrange for a home help or meals on wheels to provide food.

My father, who has dementia, can no longer cope on his own but he refuses to move out of his flat. A social worker told me that my father may be 'Sectioned'. What does this mean?

Sometimes people with dementia may behave in ways that put their own safety or the safety of others at risk. For example, your father may be leaving the gas on or wandering the streets in the middle of the night. Such behaviour is especially dangerous when someone is living alone.

If the social workers and doctors involved consider that it is no longer safe for someone with dementia to live alone, they will first try to persuade them to go into some form of care, where a closer eye could be kept on them. However, some people with dementia don't realise they have a problem and are reluctant to leave their home. Striking a balance between their safety, the safety of others and their freedom is not easy.

As a last resort, the social workers and doctors involved with someone they consider to be at risk can force that person to go into a hospital or a care home. This is the process commonly known as 'sectioning', because it uses powers under a section of the Mental Health Act (1983) for England and Wales. The terms of the section allow a person at risk to be taken to a place of safety without their consent. This is an uncommon step, which is not taken lightly. It may, however, be necessary in extreme situations.

Services for people at home

My wife has been diagnosed with Alzheimer's disease. I would like to try to care for her at home. What sort of services might be available? Will we have to pay?

The policy of community care (see p. 107) is based on an assumption that people should be helped to remain in their own homes for as long as possible if that is their wish. However, some local Health Authorities and Social Services offer more community care services than others. A person who might be able to continue to live at home with the amount of support provided in some places, might not be able to do so elsewhere. The extent to which people are expected to pay for community care services also varies from place to place. It is common for charges to be made for some services, depending on the recipient's income and savings. There may be waiting lists.

Services sometimes provided under community care are:
- home helps (see the next answer);
- meals on wheels;
- continence advice and special laundry services;
- advice on aids to increase safety in the home (see p. 78);
- equipment;
- home care (see p. 117);
- different types of nursing care (see p. 115);
- physiotherapy to help with mobility;
- chiropody;
- speech and language therapy;
- day centres (see p. 116);
- respite care (see p. 117).

Some services have to be provided wherever you live if the needs assessment (see p.108) recognises you need them. These are home helps, day centres, meals on wheels and advice on aids in the home.

Social Services are going to provide a home help because my husband has Alzheimer's disease. What sort of jobs will she do?

The type of work done by home helps varies – according to need and also according to local Social Services provisions. Your husband's care manager (see p. 108) will be able to tell you exactly what to expect. Jobs often done by home helps include light housework, shopping and cooking. Some home helps also help with aspects of personal care, such as help with getting up in the morning, getting ready for bed in the evening, and at mealtimes.

My wife has had Alzheimer's disease for some time now and I am beginning to realise that I may soon

need some more help with looking after her. What sort of nursing care might be available on the NHS, and who should I speak to?

You wife's GP or hospital specialist will be able to tell you about the nursing services that might be available to help you look after your wife. The way that community nursing services are organised – and also their availability – varies from one area to another. There may be a long waiting list.

When someone with Alzheimer's disease is living at home, various community-based nurses may become involved. The most important of these tends to be the community psychiatric nurse, often known as a CPN. These nurses work as part of a team that includes psychiatrists specialising in the care of elderly people. CPNs are sometimes involved in needs assessments (see p. 108). They may also make visits to monitor patients who have dementia and to give advice and help to carers. CPNs also liaise with other specialists about arranging respite care (see p. 117), continence advice, district nursing, support for carers, etc.

The other community-based nurse who often becomes involved when someone has Alzheimer's disease is the district nurse. District nurses, sometimes known as community nurses, have had special training in nursing people at home. They provide practical nursing care, such as changing wound dressings, supervising medication and giving injections. They may also help with tasks such as bathing, dressing and toileting, sometimes with the help of less highly qualified nursing auxiliaries, such as bath nurses. District nurses will also provide advice on equipment and aids, particularly continence aids.

Are there any specialist Alzheimer's nurses who might be able to help me?

In a very few places in London and the south of England there are specialist nurses called Admiral nurses, who are trained to look after the carers of people with Alzheimer's disease. If you want to know if there is an Admiral nurse in your area you should contact the Dementia Relief Trust (address in Appendix 1).

Day care

I am unhappy to leave my mother alone all day when I am out at work. She has Alzheimer's disease. Could she go to a day centre?

Many areas have day centres that provide day care for people with Alzheimer's disease and other dementias. Centres are run by local Health Authorities (when they may be known as a day hospital), less commonly by Social Services, and increasingly by voluntary organisations. You can find out about local day care by asking your mother's GP, speaking to Social Services or contacting local voluntary organisations, such as the Alzheimer's Disease Society or Age Concern. In some areas day care is provided by nursing homes.

Day centres can allow carers to continue to work or to have some time to themselves, while providing the person who has Alzheimer's disease with appropriate care away from home. However, the quality of day care varies. Before your mother starts attending a centre, make sure there are suitable rooms, that the staff are well trained, that there are interesting and relevant activities (see p. 72) during the day and that the food is varied and nice to eat. You should be given proper information by the day care manager about what to expect and how to complain.

Transport should be available to and from day care. Try to avoid long travelling times – more than an hour may leave people more confused and tired. A charge may be made for day care and also for transport and food.

My sister, who has dementia, refuses to go to the

**day centre. I am over eighty myself and can't cope
with her on my own all day. Might it be possible for
someone to come in and help care for her at home?**

Before making other arrangements for your sister, it would be
worth seeing if you can find out why she doesn't like the day
centre. It is possible, for example, that a change of transport,
or your accompanying her on a few occasions, or a change in
the activities provided for her at the centre could make it
more acceptable.

If the day centre really is not possible, then home care is
an alternative in many areas. Home care is sometimes called
a sitting service, but good home care is a lot more than just
sitting. A home care-worker will come into your home and
look after the person with dementia while you have a rest, do
the shopping, visit friends, have your hair done or just do
what you want to do.

Home care is usually arranged for part of a day and paid for
on an hourly basis. It is provided by Social Services, by voluntary organisations such as the Association of Crossroads
Care Attendants Schemes (see Appendix 1), and by private
agencies. Make sure that any agency you use has well-
trained staff who know about dementia. Members of the
United Kingdom Home Care Association (see Appendix 1)
have a code of practice.

Some home care agencies also take people with dementia
out, for a walk to the park, on visits or shopping. Voluntary
organisations often arrange trips out for groups.

Respite care

What is respite care and how do I get it?

Respite care is for carers. It means having someone look
after the person you are caring for to give you a break, a
respite from caring. Respite is very important for you and

the person you are caring for. If you don't have a rest or a holiday then you won't be able to go on caring. You can find out about respite care provision in your area by asking the GP or hospital consultant of the person you care for.

Respite care can take a number of forms. Usually, a person with dementia will go into a hospital or care home for a week or two. Respite beds used to be provided in many long-stay hospitals and all Health Authorities should provide some respite care. In some areas, 'home respite' is available. This means that people move into your home for a time to look after the person with dementia so that you can have a break. Private nursing homes also sometimes offer respite care if they have vacant beds. Some even do so at a reduce rate or free. This is not a bad way of trying out a nursing home which may be needed in the future.

As a carer you have a right to a carers' needs assessment (see p. 109). Ask Social Services for an assessment of your needs and request that respite care is arranged. You will probably have to pay a contribution to the cost of Social Services respite, but it is worth arguing about it as they do have discretion over this.

People with dementia may find it difficult to settle into respite care. It is a matter of trial and error and you will need to be sure that the needs of the person you care for are really understood. It may be difficult, but remember that respite is in your and their long-term interests.

I am seventy and looking after my wife who has Alzheimer's. Recently I had flu and couldn't cope. Luckily my sister came round and helped look after us both. What could I do if my sister wasn't there?

You cannot care for someone properly if you are ill yourself. If necessary, your wife could go into emergency respite care. Your social worker would be able to organise this. Most Social Service departments have special facilities for just such emergencies, and your wife could be admitted to a respite bed at very short notice.

10
Residential and nursing homes

Introduction

Most people with Alzheimer's disease and other dementias
will eventually need to go into a care home. The demands of
looking after someone with dementia day in day out over a
long period of time usually become too great for most family
carers, however much they may love the person who is ill.
A residential or nursing home can provide the best solution
for everyone. This chapter explains the difference between

residential and nursing homes. It also gives useful advice on what to look for when choosing a home and on how to make the move into the home as easy as possible.

Is a home necessary?

My husband who has dementia was taken into hospital because he has become incontinent and I cannot go on looking after him at home. The hospital now says he has to be put in a nursing home. I think he would be better cared for in hospital. Can they discharge him against my will?

Very few people with dementia are now cared for in hospital. People are usually admitted to hospital for assessment and are only kept there if they need frequent supervision by a hospital consultant or constant specialist nursing. If a person is considered not to require NHS continuing care they have no right to occupy a hospital bed. However, they do have a right to refuse to be discharged into a residential or nursing home for which they will have to pay.

Before the hospital can discharge your husband it must arrange a multi-disciplinary assessment of your husband's needs. The assessment should involve staff from the hospital, your husband's GP and also Social Services. Your husband's view, if possible, and also your view must be taken into account.

If your husband is to be returned to the community, Social Services must arrange care (see Chapter 9 for information on community care).

The hospital consultant has the final decision whether your husband should stay in hospital. There are locally agreed criteria based on national guidelines for NHS continuing care. If you are not happy about the decision you can appeal, but only if the guidelines have been incorrectly followed. You cannot appeal against the guidelines themselves.

My aunt, when she was dying of cancer, was cared for very well in a hospice. Can hospices look after people with dementia?

The hospice movement was started to provide special care for people who are dying. It has developed great expertise in controlling pain and in helping people to take control of their own deaths. Hospices are not really suitable for people with dementia, much of their skill is directed towards helping patients to make choices for themselves and to face up to their own terminal illness. At the end of their lives, people with dementia are not able to act in this way.

It is true, however, that nursing homes which care for people with dementia at the end of their lives have things to learn from the hospice movement. Respect, dignity, choice and acceptance of death are all of value to people with dementia and those who love them. The best doctors, nurses and care-workers know this and try hard to provide the right kind of care for people with dementia who are dying.

The staff in a good nursing home will be able to talk to you about how they deal with dying and the special care they give people at the end of their lives.

I did not wish to put my husband with Alzheimer's disease into a home so early on. It was hell with him at home as I still have children living here, but then it is hell seeing him in the nursing home. There is no answer or is there?

It is common to feel guilty when someone close to you has to go into a care home. You probably feel guilty because in a residential or nursing home the care is not going to be so personal and you may feel you have let your husband down. This may be made worse by reproach from your husband who probably does not understand that you simply could not manage him in your own home.

The most important way to respond to feelings of guilt is to recognise the way you feel so that you are able to make clear-headed decisions about the future and what is right for the whole family. You should also realise that nothing you did or didn't do could have prevented the disease. You cannot influence the timing or the eventual outcome of Alzheimer's disease. All you can do is to ensure that your husband is comfortable, safe and reasonably content.

Try to get along to a carers' support group. You may be surprised how many people feel as you do.

Information sources

I think the time has come to look for a nursing home for my mother who has dementia. How do I find out about nursing homes in the area where she lives?

Many GP practices have lists of local care homes and some information about them. Your Social Services department may also have such a list. However, these lists will often do no more than give the names and addresses of homes, so you will need to find out yourself which homes look after people with dementia.

The most comprehensive source of information on care homes is almost certainly the CHIC database (Care Homes Information on CD Rom). This is a computer data base that lists some 30,000 care homes, and provides basic information about them including the number of beds, specialist services and costs. It also includes information about which homes employ Alzheimer's Disease Society accredited care-workers. Quite a number of local authorities now have access to this database. If you are not able to gain access to it locally, the Alzheimer's Disease Society will send you a print-out for the town or area you need.

Another option is to contact the Elderly Accommodation Council (see Appendix 1). This organisation will send you a questionnaire to fill in and, for a small fee, will send a list of homes which might meet your requirements.

There are also various commercially produced directories, some with the support of Social Service departments. These directories contain useful information but it is important to remember that they are compiled on the basis of information from the home owners and are funded by advertising.

None of these lists or directories inspects or recommends homes. You will still have to find out for yourselves what is suitable and also what your mother can afford or Social Services will pay for. It can be very time-consuming visiting homes and trying to choose a good one, but it is usually worth the effort. Also try asking people you know if they can make any recommendations. Early planning is important because good homes are often full and there may be waiting lists.

Types of homes

What is the difference between residential homes and nursing homes, and are only nursing homes suitable for people with dementia?

The main difference between residential and nursing homes is that residential homes do not have to have nurses on the staff, whereas nursing homes must employ qualified nurses and must be able to provide 24-hour nursing care.

Not all people with dementia need to be in a nursing home. (People with dementia make up some two-thirds of all the people currently in these two types of care home.) In general, residential homes look after people who are more active and alert. Residential homes will help them with washing, dressing and toileting and of course provide meals and activities. Sometimes, a residential home will allow a person to stay on there even though they have developed dementia or become more frail. There will, however, be less nursing care than would be available in a nursing home.

People with dementia who also have physical and/or behavioural problems will need the level of care provided by a nursing home. It may also be better for people without these added problems to go straight into a nursing home, to avoid the disruption of having to move them again at a later date. Many people in nursing homes will have some dementia. Some nursing homes specialise in caring for people with dementia. People who are very difficult to care for will need to go into a specialist nursing home or to be looked after in an NHS hospital.

Who usually provides residential homes and nursing homes, and how are they regulated?

Sometimes a Local Authority has its own residential homes (sometimes called 'part III homes'). Other residential homes are provided by private organisations or individuals or on a not-for-profit basis by registered charities or religious organisations. Residential homes are registered and inspected by the local Social Services department.

Most nursing homes are privately owned by individuals or, increasingly, by big companies. Some are run by charities. Nursing homes are usually more expensive than residential homes because of the nursing care that they provide. Nursing homes must be registered with and inspected by the local Health Authority.

Some homes have dual registration as residential and nursing homes. It has been suggested that the distinction between residential and nursing home care is a false one, particularly as most older people need more care as time goes on and it is not sensible for them to have to move.

Choosing a home

My father lives alone and has Alzheimer's disease. Even with a home help he cannot manage on his own any more. What should I look for when choosing a home for him?

First you need to know that the home will take people with dementia and knows how to look after them. Your father's GP, consultant, social worker or community psychiatric nurse may be able to make suggestions, as will the nearest branch of the Alzheimer's Disease Society. When you have some names and addresses you can write or telephone to find out about the level of care provided, the fees and if a place is available. Many homes will send a brochure but you should check the facts for yourself.

If you can, make appointments to visit several homes before choosing one. Even two homes offering exactly the same level of care can have a quite different atmosphere. When you have a short-list of homes, take your father to visit them if you possibly can. After all, it will be his home and he has a right to choose as far as he is able.

Choosing a suitable home is a matter of observing carefully and asking lots of questions. Speak to the person in charge and also to members of staff. Try to assess how knowledge-able they are, especially about the needs of people with dementia. Also try to speak to other residents and their families to find out what they think about the care offered.

Some questions to consider when choosing are:
• Where is the home situated? Will it be easy for friends and family to visit?
• Are there places to get out to? Are outings arranged?
• Is there a safe garden to walk in?
• Is the home friendly, welcoming and homely?
• Is it well-furnished?
• Are there enough rooms for residents to sit in?
• Is it clean and sweet smelling? There should be no smell of urine.
• What is the home's practice about smoking?
• Are there activities going on? How are chairs arranged? Is the television just left on all day?
• Is there access for wheelchairs or walking frames? Are there suitably adapted toilets and baths?
• Can your father have a single room if that is what he would prefer?

- Can he bring his own furniture and other possessions?
- Can residents use their own rooms to be private and do staff respect their need for privacy?
- Will he have his own toilet? Are there enough toilets and bathrooms for all the residents?
- Do the staff treat people with tact and respect when helping them with bathing or visiting the toilet?
- What is the food like? Is the food at the home appealing and nutritious? Are choices offered at meal-times? Does the home cater for special diets? What we eat and when we eat it is an important factor in quality of life.
- Will your father be able to eat in his room if he wishes?
- Will he be able to eat at a different time, or have a snack, just like in his own home?
- What are the arrangements for medical care?
- Are dental treatment and chiropody available?

If you feel that you need more detailed advice on choosing a home, further information is available from Age Concern, the Alzheimer's Disease Society, Counsel and Care and the Relatives Association (addresses in Appendix 1).

Do the staff running a care home have to be properly qualified? How can I find out if they are trained to do the job?

All care homes have to be registered, either with Social Services or with the Health Authority (see p. 124). All nursing homes are required to have a qualified nurse on duty at all times, but apart from this there are no requirements for care homes to be owned by or to employ qualified staff.

When choosing a care home, you should ask the owner or manager what qualifications they or other senior staff have and what arrangements are made for staff training. You should also make a point of asking if they have particular knowledge of looking after people with dementia. Apart from general nursing qualifications, psychiatric nursing or social work qualifications are relevant. It would also be useful to know if there is an occupational therapist either on the staff or coming into the home regularly. The home should have its own training programme for care staff, for instance staff might follow the Alzheimer's Disease Society care learning programme and be ADS accredited care-workers.

You can tell a lot from the way staff in a home behave. Are they sensitive, tolerant and caring as well as efficient, hard-working and capable? Good care is a matter of natural ability as well as training.

Making the move

It must be very upsetting to have to move from your own home into a care home. What is the best way of preparing for this and arranging it so that my mother is distressed as little as possible?

Good planning and preparation is the best way of minimising distress for people when they move. Often people go into a care home when there is a crisis and that makes things more difficult for everyone. It is important to face up in advance to the likelihood that residential or nursing home care will be needed eventually.

Find out about the suitable homes in your area and visit them all. Take your mother with you if she is able. It will be her home, so as far as possible she should choose. It might help if your mother could go to a home for day care, perhaps one day a week or more for a while, so that she can see if she likes it and get used to the people.

Another possibility might be for your mother to take advantage of a home's respite break provision and go and stay there for a week occasionally. This can have benefits for all concerned. Your mother will become familiar with the people and the place, you will know whether or not she likes it, and the staff will find out about her needs. A series of short stays of this kind, preparing for a permanent move, will also help you to discover if the care in the home is good.

It's not always possible to do as much preparation as this but do try to make sure that your mother visits different homes and has some choice.

It will be helpful if you can visit your mother often when she first moves into the home, and do try to make sure she knows when you will be returning. Also make sure that she has some of her own furniture and some familiar objects, such as ornaments and photographs, with her.

This can be a very distressing and difficult time for everyone, but handled well it will bring security for your mother and a sense of release for you as a carer.

Privacy or company?

It seems to me to be quite wrong that my sister, who has Alzheimer's disease, is put in a room by herself in the nursing home. She can hardly communicate and she needs company. I think she would benefit from sharing a room with other people.

Everyone is different, but it is thought to be better for most people in nursing homes to have their own bedrooms rather than needing to share with a stranger. Having your own bedroom means that privacy and dignity can be maintained at all times, particularly when intimate care and personal tasks are involved.

Having your own bedroom shouldn't mean you are alone. People should be out of bed and staff should be talking to them and involving them as far as is possible in the life of the care home. If you think your sister is just being left alone in bed for long periods, then the home is not caring for her very well. You should speak to the home manager if you think this is the case.

Obviously there are a few people who like company so much that they enjoy being with others all the time. Shared rooms are very often provided in homes, usually at a lower cost, and if you are sure that this is what your sister would like, even though she is now ill, you should be able to arrange it.

Possible ill treatment

My father is in a home. He has severe dementia and must be quite a handful. The last couple of times I have visited him I have noticed bruises on his arms. The staff all seem very nice but I'm worried someone may be hitting him. What should I do?

People with dementia may have bruises for a number of reasons. Older people have fragile skin that tends to bruise with little pressure. Your father may be unsteady on his feet and bump into things or fall. He may have become involved in an altercation with another resident. However, older people are at risk from ill treatment or neglect by a care-worker.

If you suspect that your father is being ill treated in the home, there are several things you should do. First, try to see as much as possible of your father's skin (you could say you want to bath him) and look for bruises elsewhere. Also, glance at other residents to see whether anyone else has bruises. If you are still concerned, write down the dates of your visits and the location of your father's bruises. You should then take this information with you and ask the home manager for an explanation. If the home manager fails to provide you with a satisfactory reply, you should speak to your father's social worker or to the council department that is responsible for licensing care homes.

In cases of suspected ill treatment it can be tempting to say nothing, for fear of causing more problems. However, if any ill treatment is taking place it should be investigated. Ultimately, you may feel that your father is best moved to another home, perhaps one where the staff are better trained and supervised.

Visiting

My wife is now in a nursing home because of her Alzheimer's disease. I try to visit her every day but I am finding this quite exhausting. Do you think it matters if I do not visit her quite so often?

You have probably found it very difficult to accept that you cannot look after your wife any more at home. You may feel that you have let her down and you are perhaps blaming yourself for not being able to manage. The care your wife is receiving in the nursing home will not, of course, be as personal and may not be as good as the care you were giving her at home. Many carers want to go on helping as much as they possibly can. It will probably take you a while to come to terms with the fact that your wife is quite well cared for in the home and does seem fairly content and comfortable when you visit.

Your wife is very unlikely to remember exactly when you last visited. You and your wife will enjoy your visits much more if you are less tired and more cheerful, and it sounds as if you could do with taking a break and putting trust in the people who are now looking after your wife. You will probably find it helpful to talk with one or two of the staff about how you are feeling and tell them that you are going to visit less often.

11
Legal and financial advice

Introduction

Nearly all people with Alzheimer's disease and other dementias will become unable to manage their financial affairs, and many of the people caring for them will become involved in financial or legal problems of some kind. Most of the real difficulties can be avoided or reduced by early planning. Many financial benefits are available from the state for people with dementia and their carers. However, the rules are complicated and you should seek individual advice. Also note that benefits and amounts often change, so the information given here can only be a general guide.

Remember too that if you are managing someone else's finances you should always try to involve them as much as possible. People with dementia can still make choices even if they are no longer sure of the value of things, and it is right that they should understand as much as possible of what is being decided for them.

Getting advice

Where can I get advice on legal and financial matters?

Legal and financial problems can be complicated and it is always wise to seek independent advice.

Your local Citizens Advice Bureau (CAB) is often the best starting point. Advice is free and confidential and the CAB staff will help to sort out your problems and give you clear information. Some CABx have specialist legal and financial advisors. The address of the local CAB should be in the Phone Book. If you need specifically legal advice, Law Centres give free advice on problems such as welfare rights, benefits, housing and employment. To find out of there is a Law Centre near you, ask at your local library or contact the Law Centres Federation (address in Appendix 1).

If you are arranging a will (see p. 133) or an Enduring Power of Attorney (see p. 134), you may wish to contact a solicitor. It may be helpful to ask for a recommendation from friends or relatives locally. The Alzheimer's Disease Society (address in Appendix 1) has a list of recommended solicitors who have specialist knowledge of the legal problems of people with dementia and their carers. If you are going to a solicitor for the first time do not be afraid to ask for a clear written estimate of costs and an explanation of the work they will do on your behalf.

Information on benefits can be obtained from your local Social Services department. There is also a Benefits Enquiry Line (see Appendix 1). This is a free national telephone advice and information service for people with disabilities and their carers. It provides general advice on benefits but will not answer questions on your specific situation.

Advice on benefits is also available from Age Concern, the Alzheimer's Disease Society and Alzheimer Scotland (see Appendix 1).

Legal safeguards

I have recently been diagnosed with Alzheimer's disease and I want to make a will. Are there any special things I should think about?

It is very important to make a will. It is usually easy and not expensive. Making a will makes sure that your estate goes to those you want it to and makes it much easier to settle your affairs after you die.

If your estate is only small and your plans are simple, a postal will-making service may be adequate. However, for most people, it is best to take legal advice when making a will. Always ask in advance for an estimate of the cost of making a will. Legal advice can be obtained from a Law Centre or from a solicitor. The Alzheimer's Disease Society has a list of solicitors who have a special interest and knowledge in legal matters affecting people with dementia.

When planning your will, you will need to consider your personal circumstances, your relatives and friends. If you own your own house and share it with someone who is caring for you, you may want to make arrangements to protect their interest in it. You may also want to plan for nursing home fees in the future. It is not easy to think about the difficulties ahead, but if you can manage to do this and take good advice you will help not only yourself but those you love.

Many solicitors offer to draw up an Enduring Power of Attorney (see below) at the same time as making a will and have an all-inclusive price. You may think this is a good idea.

What is an Enduring Power of Attorney?

An Enduring Power of Attorney (EPA) is a legal document in which one person gives another or others the power to handle his or her financial affairs. This power can only be given when the person giving it is mentally capable of understanding what he or she is doing. For this reason, it is important for anyone who has been given a diagnosis of dementia to consider having an Enduring Power of Attorney drawn up as soon as possible. A doctor's advice may be sought if there is any doubt about a person's mental capacity.

An Enduring Power of Attorney will give the recipient considerable power over the donor's money, so it is important to choose someone that the donor trusts and who is capable of making judgements in his or her interests. Usually a husband or wife choose each other or one of their children. It is possible to appoint joint attorneys.

An Enduring Power of Attorney is made on a special form which you can get from a law stationer or solicitor. The form allows the donor to specify the powers that the attorney will have. It names the person appointed as attorney and must be signed by the attorney, the donor and at least one witness who is not a relative of the donor. It is important to use the right form and to complete it properly, otherwise the attorneyship will be invalid. An Enduring Power of Attorney should not be confused with an ordinary Power of Attorney, which ceases to be valid when a person becomes mentally incapacitated.

When the attorney believes that the donor has become mentally incapable he or she must notify the donor and certain close relatives of his or her intention to register the Enduring Power of Attorney. An application to register must be made to the Public Trust Office (see Appendix 1). The registration will take several weeks because the Office must hold the papers for 35 days to allow objections. Registration will cost around £50 (1998) if you do it yourself. If you use a solicitor to register the Enduring Power of Attorney for you it could cost several hundred pounds. If all is in order, notice of approval is sent and the attorney is then able to act in accordance with the terms laid down by the donor.

My father has had dementia for two years. Can he still make a will or sign an Enduring Power of Attorney?

It may still be possible depending on your father's mental capabilities. If you are worried about your father's competence, to avoid problems in future, it may be wise to consult a doctor or solicitor to ensure your father still has 'testamentary capacity'. People's mental competence may change, so it may be possible when seeking consent to choose a time when your father is most alert.

For a will to be valid, your father will need to be able to understand what a will is, be aware of the size of his estate and be aware of the individuals who may have a claim to the estate. In order to sign an Enduring Power of Attorney, your father also needs to understand, at that time, that he is giving power to manage his affairs to another.

Financial incompetence

My widowed mother has always been a methodical and well-organised person and doesn't like me to interfere in her financial affairs. However, she is getting forgetful and her electricity was nearly turned off because she didn't pay the bill. What can I do?

A good way of ensuring that your mother's bills are paid on time would be to suggest that she signs direct debit forms for her utility bills and for any other regular payments, such as rent. If she won't sign a direct debit, perhaps she would find a regular payment by standing order more acceptable.

Most utility companies – water, gas and electricity – have a register of older customers and those with special needs, and you should inform them that your mother may not respond in time. All utility companies will have a code of practice covering any cutting off of the supply, and copies should be available. The various companies will probably agree to inform you if they have a problem with your mother's bills. You should prepare yourself for the likelihood that your mother's ability to manage her affairs will get worse.

My father, who has Alzheimer's disease, is no longer able to manage his money safely. He forgets to get his pension, loses cash and refuses to pay for things in shops. What can we do?

It is usual for people to lose their understanding of money as Alzheimer's disease progresses. There are a number of practical things that you can do to keep your father independent for as long as possible while protecting his money.

One thing you can do is to make arrangements concerning your father's pension. For example, it may be possible for someone to be authorised to collect it for him. If the local Benefits Agency are contacted they would put that person's name in the order book. The person chosen is known as the 'authorised agent'. However, your father cannot make a valid choice if he does not understand what he is doing. In this case, appointeeship should be considered. This is a more formal arrangement and should be made through the Benefits Agency. Alternatively, if your father has a bank or building society account, you can make an arrangement for his pension to be paid directly into that.

If you have an Enduring Power of Attorney (see p. 134), you could use it to restrict your father's access to cash. If you don't have an EPA, you or someone else will need to apply to become his receiver. However, be careful. If you don't have an EPA, the bank may refuse to deal with you and may take action to freeze your father's account on the grounds of his mental incapacity.

If your father is known in the local shops, you may feel able to explain to the shopkeepers and make arrangements with them to pay for goods if he refuses to do so. If your father has a helpful bank or building society manager, it may be wise to speak to them so that they can alert you if your father takes out more money than he should need. Many people with dementia lose or hide money. If possible, you should limit the amount of cash that your father has at any time, and should try to ensure that bills and regular payments, such as for gas, electricity or rent, are paid by standing order or direct debit.

My husband has always looked after our money. He used to be so well-organised and paid all the bills. He was very unwilling to hand over to me as he became more forgetful. Now he cannot even write a cheque. How can I or our son take over his finances?

If your husband is able to grant you an Enduring Power of Attorney (see p. 134), you should take steps to arrange this at once. This is the simplest arrangement.

However, if your husband is not capable of granting an EPA (see p. 135), and you live in England or Wales, you will have to apply to the Court of Protection (see Appendix 1) to become his receiver. (Different arrangements apply in Scotland and in Northern Ireland. Alzheimer Scotland or the Alzheimer's Disease Society could advise you on this.)

The Court of Protection is an office of the Supreme Court. It exists to protect the property and finances of people who are mentally unable to manage their own affairs. The Court of Protection will consider the medical evidence about your husband, as well as the details of his financial position and that of his family. Having considered the evidence, the Court then usually appoints a close relative as receiver. If you become your husband's receiver, you will be able to take over his bank account and pay bills and receive income on his behalf as long as you try to act in his best interests. You will be accountable to the Court of Protection for what you do.'

Once you have been appointed receiver, the administration is handled by the Public Trust Office (see Appendix 1). It will charge a fee when you are appointed receiver and will require you to provide an annual account of how your husband's money has been spent. There will be an annual fee for administration. Having to go to the Court of Protection to obtain receivership is time consuming and expensive. Many carers feel very unhappy about this system but it must be remembered that it is designed to protect the person who is mentally incapacitated.

Benefits

Are there any financial benefits that are available to help people with Alzheimer's disease?

There are several ways that you can get financial help from the state if you are caring for someone with a dementia such as Alzheimer's disease. There is no benefit that relates to people with dementia specifically. The benefits system can be rather confusing and you may find it helpful to seek advice. Your social worker should be able to help you, or your local Citizens Advice Bureau. There is also a freephone Benefits Enquiry Line (see Appendix 1) for people with disabilities, including people with dementia. The Alzheimer's Disease Society (see Appendix 1) has a useful information sheet on Welfare benefits which provides more detail than can be included here.

All benefits depend in some way on individual financial or personal circumstances. It is best to check out as many different benefits as possible. Some depend on income, others on age and others on the reason, such as illness or unemployment, that help is needed.

All people with dementia should be able to apply for either Attendance Allowance or Disability Living Allowance to help them with their care needs. These benefits do not depend on income or savings and are tax free. Nor do they take account of where a person lives or if they live alone or with a carer. People whose care needs develop before the age of 65 should apply for Disability Living Allowance. People aged 65 and over should apply for the Attendance Allowance. Both allowances are paid at different rates depending on needs. The Disability Living Allowance has a mobility payment as well as a care payment.

Either allowance can be paid to people who need help with daily care such as washing, dressing, eating, toileting and taking medication. They can also be paid if people need supervision to avoid risks when inside or outside the home. People who have dementia will qualify for different rates of the various allowances depending on their needs. Since dementia is a progressive illness, it is important to reapply as needs change.

People under the age of 65 who have difficulty walking may apply for the mobility component of the Disability Living Allowance. There are two rates. A lower rate is paid to people who show that although they are able to walk they need guidance to stop them getting lost. The higher rate is paid to people who are unable to walk due to paralysis or weakness or whose walking is severely limited.

Forms for applying for the various allowances are available from the Post Office.

My husband had to leave his job because he became forgetful and inefficient. He was later diagnosed as having dementia. What financial help can we get? Will his pension rights be affected?

There can be problems for people with dementia who have to give up work or are sacked because of undiagnosed dementia. People may have lost unemployment benefits or sick pay or pension rights. It is important to inform your husband's former employers of the diagnosis and to ask for his rights to be protected. If your husband was a member of a union or staff association, they may be able to help.

People with dementia who have had to give up work and are below retirement age may be able to apply for Incapacity Benefit or Severe Disablement Allowance.

Incapacity Benefit may be claimed if someone is unable to work because of illness or disability and is not entitled to statutory sick pay. The person claiming the benefit must have paid sufficient National Insurance contributions. Incapacity Benefit is paid at three rates: a lower rate for the first 28 weeks, another rate for the remainder of the first year, and a long-term rate after one year. People getting the higher rate Disability Living Allowance can get the long-term rate of Incapacity Benefit after 28 weeks. Incapacity Benefit is not affected by your husband's income or savings but may be taxed. The long-term rate is taxable.

Severe Disablement Allowance is payable to people who have been unable to work for 28 weeks because of their disability but cannot claim Incapacity Benefit because they have not paid enough National Insurance contributions. Only people under 65 can claim this benefit. It is not taxed but may not be payable if certain other Social Security benefits are already being received.

My wife was only 49 when she developed Alzheimer's disease. We managed for a few years on my income after she stopped work. Now I have had to give up working to care for her so we have very little to live on. Are there any benefits to help carers?

You should be able to apply for the Invalid Care Allowance. This can be paid to carers who spend at least 35 hours a week looking after someone. The person they look after must be getting either the Attendance Allowance or the Disability Living Allowance at the middle or higher rate. So if your wife is not claiming one of these you should apply for them first.

Carers can claim if they are over 16 years old but under pensionable age. Payment does not depend on previous National Insurance contributions. Indeed, this benefit will give you class 1 National Insurance contribution credits to help protect your pension rights when you reach 65. Invalid Care Allowance is taxable.

If your income is low and your savings are below the limit set by the government, you may also be able to claim Income Support. This is paid to people on low incomes to help them with basic living expenses. Income Support can be paid in full or as a top-up to other benefits or pensions. Attendance Allowance or Disability Living Allowance are ignored when calculating a person's entitlement to Income Support.

If you are entitled to Income Support, you are also likely to qualify for Housing Benefit and Council Tax Benefit and also for free prescriptions and other NHS benefits. Your social worker or local Citizens Advice Bureau should be able to help you work out all the help you and your wife can get.

My mother has come to live with me so I can care for her. Do I have to pay the full Council Tax now? I used to get the single person's discount.

Your Council Tax is set and collected by your Local Authority and you should contact them about possible discounts and how to claim them. (People who live in Northern Ireland, where there is still a rating system, should contact the rebate section of the local rate collection agency.) It is likely that you will still qualify for the single person's discount of 25% on your Council Tax bill.

Your mother will be 'disregarded' for the purposes of Council Tax assessment if you are caring for her for at least 35 hours a week and if she is receiving the highest rate of the Disability Living Allowance or Attendance Allowance. (Note that this exemption does not apply when a carer is looking after a husband, wife, partner or child under 18).

Even if you are still working, you can ask for your mother to be 'disregarded' for Council Tax purposes if she has a medical certificate stating that she is severely mentally impaired and is receiving the highest rate of the Disability Living Allowance or Attendance Allowance.

If your mother still has her own home, it will be exempt from Council Tax while it is empty because she has moved so that you can care for her.

If you need to extend your home by adding an extra room or bathroom because of your mother's disability, you may be able to get a reduction in the Council Tax band. Ask your Council for details of the 'Disability Reduction'.

My husband, who is only 59, has Alzheimer's disease. Can I get free prescriptions and other help for him?

Your husband has not yet reached the statutory retirement age and so is not entitled to free medical prescriptions on the grounds of age. However, he will qualify for free prescriptions and other NHS benefits if he is receiving Income Support or Disability Living Allowance and has savings of less than £8,000 (1998). Even if he does not meet these criteria, it might still be worth applying if his income is low.

Other NHS benefits include free dental treatment from NHS dentists, free sight tests and vouchers towards glasses, and free hearing tests and hearing aids. You should also be able to get free continence aids and vouchers for aids such as wheelchairs. Help with travel costs for NHS hospital visits is also available. Ask for claim forms from your husband's GP, the practice nurse or at the hospital.

I have been turned down for the benefit I applied for. How can I appeal?

If you think you have been turned down unfairly for a benefit, you have a right to disagree with the decision. Write to the office that made the decision and ask them to review it. Give them additional or correct information if you think they have not taken all the facts into account. If they do not change their decision you may be able to apply to an independent appeal tribunal.

You can also appeal if you think you have not been awarded the correct rate of a benefit, such as the lower or higher rate of the Attendance Allowance or the mobility part of the Disability Living Allowance.

Appealing can be complicated and the rules are different for different benefits, so get advice as soon as possible from a Citizens Advice Bureau, your local council Welfare Rights office, the freephone Benefits Enquiry Line or the Alzheimer's Disease Society (see Appendix 1 for addresses and telephone numbers).

My wife has Alzheimer's disease and I have retired early to care for her. Can I get grants or financial help from anywhere other than the Benefits Agency?

There are various organisations that may be able to help you with particular bills, items of equipment or respite breaks. Many religious communities offer help to their members. If you or the person you care for belong to a trade union or a benevolent or friendly society then they may be able to help. There are also trusts and charities specially to help people connected with the armed forces or who have worked in a particular trade or profession. A number of local and national charities make small grants to people in need.

Whether or not you can get help will depend on the rules of the organisation you apply to, what funds are available and what your needs are. You can only find out by making contact with particular organisations.

One directory that might be of use to you is 'A Guide to Grants for Individuals in Need'. This lists many sources of help and tells you how to apply. It is published by the Directory of Social Change and should be in your local library.

Your social worker or doctor or local religious group may know about local charities or sources of help.

The national Alzheimer's Disease Society (see Appendix 1) has a caring fund. Grants of up to £500 (1998) are available to help with daily living, transport, respite or temporary financial need. An application form is available from the

Society. Your local Alzheimer's Disease Society branch may give small grants or arrange respite breaks.

My husband went into hospital for an assessment but while he was there he got worse and now it seems unlikely he will be able to come home. What happens to his Attendance Allowance and other benefits?

Your husband's Attendance Allowance will be suspended after he has been in hospital for 28 days. If he has a state retirement pension, this will be reduced after he has been in hospital for six weeks. The amount by which it will be reduced will depend on your husband's actual circumstances. Other benefits, if he is receiving any, may also be affected.

If your husband is discharged from hospital into a care home, new financial arrangements will need to be made. If his fees are to be paid for by Social Services or by the NHS, Attendance Allowance will stop but your husband will be expected to claim all the other benefits he is entitled to. Most of the benefit money will go towards paying the home's fees, but your husband will be entitled to a small sum for personal spending each week. If your husband is paying his own care home fees, he can continue to claim and receive the Attendance Allowance.

Paying for home fees

Some people in my area who have dementia are cared for free of charge in hospital, but I have been told I have to find a care home for my father. Why do some people get NHS care and others have to go private?

Government policies during the 1980s and 1990s encouraged local Health Authorities to reduce the number of hospital beds available for people with dementia. It was argued that there was no need for the NHS to provide care for most dementia sufferers because most of them are not really ill. They might need social and nursing care, but they do not generally need medical care. Obviously not everyone agrees with this argument. The government has set up a Royal Commission on Long-term Care to look at all the issues.

Your local Health Authority must publish its criteria for NHS continuing care. These 'eligibility criteria' set out the conditions that must be met if the NHS is to provide long-term care for someone with dementia. Usually it will only be when someone needs constant nursing care and regular supervision by a hospital consultant by reason of extreme frailty or severe mental disturbance.

If you look at the eligibility criteria in your area and think that your father meets them, you can ask his consultant to admit him to an NHS bed. If the hospital won't accept him, you can ask for a review. However, the review will only look at whether the eligibility criteria have been properly applied, not at whether they are fair in the first place.

Although my mother has fairly substantial savings she does not own her own home. She receives the state widow's pension. Will she have to pay for all her nursing home care?

Your mother will have to pay for her own nursing home care if she has savings of more than £16,000 (1998). Her state widow's pension is unlikely to cover more than a small proportion of the fees, so she will have to find the rest of the money from her savings.

If your mother has enough money to pay for nursing home fees for the foreseeable future, you and she can make your own choice of home and financial arrangements. However, if you choose a very luxurious and expensive home, your mother will probably have to move to a cheaper home approved by Social Services if her money ever runs out.

If you think that your mother's savings are not likely to cover her home fees indefinitely, it would be wise to ask Social Services to conduct a needs assessment (see p. 108) before you find her a home. If the assessment confirms that your mother does need to go into a home, Social Services will specify the amount that they will pay as and when your mother's savings are reduced to £16,000.

If you are not able to get a Social Services assessment before your mother goes into a home, you should check whether the home's fees fall within the limits laid down by Social Services. If they do, you should make arrangements with Social Services to assess your mother's needs well before her savings fall to the level that will qualify her for financial help.

Social Services are making arrangements for my wife to be moved into a nursing home. They are making a financial assessment of her income and savings and have asked me to tell them about my money as well. Is this right?

The local authority can only assess the financial resources of the person who is receiving care. They do not have the power to insist that you provide details of your income or savings. The local authority has to work out your wife's contribution to her care costs based on her finances. They have a duty to make up the difference, if any, between the cost of the nursing home and her contribution.

However, the 1948 National Assistance Act (section 42) states that husbands and wives are liable to support each other financially. This is one of the 'liable relative rules' and only applies to married couples. Your local authority can ask you to make a contribution but has no power to insist that you reveal details of your finances to them. Normally a husband or wife can make an offer of an amount that he or she thinks it reasonable to pay towards the cost of caring for their spouse. Age Concern (see Appendix 1) has produced a factsheet covering the liable relative rules: Paying for Care in a Residential & Nursing Home if you have a partner (Factsheet No. 5).

I have cared for my husband, who has Alzheimer's disease, for a number of years now but recently I have been ill myself and we have reluctantly decided he should go into a nursing home. He has an occupational pension as well as his state retirement pension, and we have savings of about £20,000. It seems he will have to pay his own care home fees but this leave me with very little to live on. Is there anything I can do?

It can be very hard on one partner when a husband or wife goes into a nursing home and pays their own fees out of what was before shared income and savings.

Your savings, if they are in a joint bank account, will be divided equally between you. So £10,000 will be treated as yours. The other £10,000 must be used to pay towards your husband's fees if his income doesn't cover the full amount. When he has less than £8,000 savings, Social Services may make up the difference. It may be worth splitting your accounts so that your husband is means-tested separately.

You will continue to receive the married woman's pension. You may also claim half of your husband's occupational pension. If this is a very small amount, however, you may be better off not claiming it and applying for Income Support. If you get Income Support you will also be able to get Housing Benefit and various NHS benefits (see p. 142).

My husband has become incontinent and I really can't cope with looking after him any more. It seems that a nursing home is the only choice now but he only has a small pension. Will I have to sell our house to pay the home fees? And what money will I have to live on?

You will not have to sell the house while you continue to live in it. You should ask Social Services to assess your husband's need for a nursing home. Then you can choose a home from the list which Social Services should give you. Social Services will make arrangements to pay your husband's fees directly to the home. His state pension will go towards the cost of the nursing home. If he has an occupational pension you can claim half of that. If he has no occupational pension and you have no pension of your own, you will be left with only the married woman's pension, which is not much to live on. You may be entitled to Income Support.

While you live in the house, Social Services will not ask you to sell it to pay for your husband's fees. However, if you stop living in it because you move or you die, they can make a claim against the proceeds of the sale. If your husband owns the house, all the value will be taken into account. If it is jointly owned, then half of it will be considered his.

I moved in with my father after my mother died. I have cared for him for many years but now he has had to go into a nursing home. I always thought that the house would be mine. It is left to me in his will but now it seems that Social Services will take it to pay for his care. Is this right?

All your father's income and savings and assets over £10,000 (usually including the house) will be taken into account when Social Services work out how much he has to contribute to the cost of the nursing home. Social Services may disregard the value of the house in some circumstances and you should ask them if they are willing to do so. In certain circumstances they must disregard it, for instance if the relative living in it is over 60 years old or is disabled.

As long as you continue to live in the house, Social Services are unlikely take it from you or sell it. They can apply for a court order to force you to sell the house but this is very rare. If you remain in the house, they may later make a charge against it for whatever amount they have contributed to your father's nursing home costs. This amount will only be payable if you decide to move and sell the house. When your father dies, the house will be yours but there may still be a charge against your father's estate if you decide to sell it.

12
Treatment

Introduction

Although there is no cure for Alzheimer's disease or for most other types of dementia, it is possible to help people with dementia, and their carers, in a variety of ways. Many of the problems associated with dementia, such as restlessness and depression, can be treated. It may also be possible, especially in the early stages of dementia, to improve someone's memory with medication or by using other methods.

People with dementia may also develop other, unrelated illnesses that require treatment.

Treatment possibilities

Is Alzheimer's disease curable?

Unfortunately, there is no cure for Alzheimer's disease at the present time. Nor can a cure be expected in the foreseeable future. Researchers are still at the stage of developing drugs that will slow down the progression of the disease, at least in some cases. They still do not know how to prevent the disease from occurring, how to stop its progression, or how to reverse its effects. It is hoped that more research into the causes of Alzheimer's disease will eventually make a cure possible, but at the present time Alzheimer's disease is incurable.

Are any forms of dementia curable?

Some of the rarer forms of dementia – for example, those associated with thyroid problems, brain tumours, obstruction to the flow of fluid through the brain, vitamin deficiencies and infections – can be cured, or helped considerably, by appropriate treatment. Sometimes the treatment is simple – such as thyroid hormone supplements to treat dementia caused by under-activity of the thyroid gland, or vitamin supplements if the problem is due to a vitamin deficiency.

Most types of dementia, however, cannot be cured and those that can be cured are very rare. The possibility that a person may be suffering from a curable type of dementia will be investigated whenever dementia is diagnosed. There is no evidence that thyroid hormone or vitamin supplements are helpful for people with dementia who do not have a deficiency of these substances. Indeed, the inappropriate use of such supplements can sometimes be harmful.

I get so frustrated. I keep coming across stories about new treatments for Alzheimer's disease, but nothing seems to be available for my wife. Why is this?

It can certainly be very frustrating to read or hear about new treatments only to find out later that they are not actually available. This is especially true when someone, like you, has a personal reason for hoping that a cure may soon be found.

The best advice is to treat all media reports with caution. Millions of people in the world want news of treatments for Alzheimer's disease. So when scientists find a treatment that appears to work, their research is often widely publicised. The problem is that after early experiments have shown that a treatment may work, many more years of research are needed to make sure that it is both effective and safe. All too often, follow-up research shows that a treatment does not work after all or that it has dangerous side effects.

New drugs for treating Alzheimer's disease have attracted a lot of publicity recently. These drugs have been found to relieve some of the symptoms of Alzheimer's disease in some people. However, they are not a cure and they are not usually effective for more than a few months. Also, they are probably effective only early in the disease, and even then may not always be useful. Many other drugs will soon be available.

Can anything halt or slow down the mental deterioration that occurs in Alzheimer's disease?

Alzheimer's disease is usually relentlessly progressive, leading to death between five and 10 years after diagnosis in most cases. However, it is often possible to slow down the rate at which the disease progresses.

One possibility may be to use an anticholinesterase drug (see page 156 for more information).

The progression of Alzheimer's disease is also likely to be slowed if good general health can be maintained. A well-balanced diet and regular exercise are important for this. Various simple measures may also contribute by protecting the so-called 'cerebral reserve'. This term refers to brain cells that can take over the function of other brain cells that die. Each individual's cerebral reserve is huge at birth but declines dramatically with age. The decline is particularly marked in people with dementias, such as Alzheimer's disease. Factors that are believed to cause a decline in the cerebral reserve include drinking alcohol, smoking, receiving blows to the head and suffering from severe infections. It makes good sense to keep all these risks to a minimum when someone has an already reduced cerebral reserve because of a dementia.

A person's physical surroundings are also important – a safe and familiar environment will help reduce confusion and may reduce the risk of a fall.

My wife has vascular dementia. Can anything help to stop things getting worse?

It may be possible to slow down the development of vascular dementia (see p.19) by treating the underlying problem, which is cerebrovascular disease (narrowing of the arteries causing reduced blood supply to the brain).

Smoking is known to thicken the blood and to increase the risk of a stroke. Anyone who has vascular dementia and smokes should consider giving up smoking.

In some cases, the doctor will prescribe drugs, such as aspirin, to thin the blood and decrease the risk of stroke. Any irregularity of the heartbeat will also be treated, as this condition also increases the risk of stroke.

If the arteries leading to the brain have become furred up by deposits known as plaques, it may be possible to perform an operation to strip away the plaques, thus widening the diameter of the artery and improving the blood supply to the brain. However, this operation has risks and is only appropriate in special circumstances. Your wife's doctor will advise you if the operation might be suitable for your wife.

If your wife's vacular dementia is accompanied by high blood pressure, this will need careful treatment. A person with cerebrovascular disease may need a relatively high blood pressure to ensure that there is an adequate supply of blood to the brain. However, if the blood pressure is very high it will need to be treated.

Dealing with doctors

As the carer doing all the work I feel I should be kept fully informed about my father's illness. But my father's doctor says he is bound by confidentiality and cannot discuss the details with me.

It is true that a doctor's relationship is directly with his or her patient and not with the patient's relative or partner. This does seem strange sometimes when the person who is ill is not able to understand what is happening to them or to give informed consent. Doctors dealing with someone with dementia usually recognise this and involve the carer in the discussions and decisions. But a carer does not have a legal right to know or to be involved.

If you have not already done so, try to explain to your father's doctor how important it is that you know what is going on. If the doctor is still unwilling to involve you, there are a number of things you can do:

- Ask your father if you can stay with him when he sees the doctor. If your father consents to your being there the doctor will probably not refuse.
- Try talking to other health professionals, such as the practice nurse or the community psychiatric nurse.
- If it is your father's hospital specialist who is being uncommunicative try talking about the problem with the GP, or vice versa.

The Law Commission has recently proposed that the law be changed to allow someone to appoint a 'Health Care Proxy'. This person would be legally involved in making decisions about the health care of someone who was mentally unable to do make his or her own decisions. This change in the law has not yet been made.

My mother, who is in a nursing home because of dementia, has been put on sedative drugs. I'm not happy with this. Shouldn't I have been consulted?

Yes, you should have been consulted. Research suggests that sedative drugs are sometimes over-used, especially in care homes. If you are unhappy about your mother's treatment, ask the manager of the home if you can see the home's doctor.

Seeing a specialist

My husband has recently been diagnosed as having Alzheimer's disease. The diagnosis was made by our GP. Should my husband now see a specialist?

General practitioners (GPs) can often diagnose Alzheimer's disease without needing to refer the patient to a specialist. It is usual for many GPs to refer a patient on to a specialist only if they are not sure about the diagnosis, or if they think that the case is not a clear-cut one.

If the GP does decide to ask for a second opinion, he may request this from a geriatrician (a doctor who specialises in physical illnesses in older people) or from a psychiatrist with a particular interest in the mental problems of older people. The GP may occasionally refer someone with dementia to a psychologist (a specialist in mental processes, such as memory) or neurologist (a doctor who specialises in nervous diseases).

A GP is able to refer people to Social Services for a needs assessment (see p. 108) so they can receive appropriate care and support. However, some Social Services departments require the opinion of a specialist before they will proceed. Your husband's GP will know what is necessary in your area. (See Chapter 9 for more information about community care).

Drug treatments

If drugs can't cure Alzheimer's disease, what can they do for someone who has it?

It is true that, as yet, no drugs have been discovered that can cure Alzheimer's disease. However, it does seem that new drugs, called cholinesterase inhibitors or anticholinesterase drugs, can slow down the progression of the disease in some cases. (See page 156 for more information.)

Other kinds of drugs are sometimes useful for controlling some of the symptoms of Alzheimer's disease, such as sleeplessness and agitation. In general, however, the use of drugs such as sleeping pills or tranquillisers should be kept to a minimum if someone has Alzheimer's disease, as they can cause increased confusion. Drugs can also be used to treat constipation, but dietary measures are generally preferable (see page 58).

A person with Alzheimer's disease may need drugs to treat other illnesses that might develop, such as a chest or urinary infection, or longer term medical conditions, such as high blood pressure or some types of heart problem.

My father is taking various kinds of pills, but he seems to be getting more and more confused. Might the drugs he is taking be making his Alzheimer's disease worse rather than better?

It is possible that some of your father's pills may be making him more confused. If you tell your father's doctor about your worry, he or she may be able to improve matters by adusting your father's medication.

In general, it is best for people with Alzheimer's disease to take as few drugs as possible, because certain types of drugs do have side effects that can make confusion worse. However, the drugs that can cause confusion unfortunately include tranquillising medication, which may, nonetheless, sometimes need to be given to people with dementia.

I have heard that there are some new drug treatments for Alzheimer's disease. What are these new drugs, what can they do, and are they available in the UK?

Worldwide there is an immense amount of research into new drug treatments for Alzheimer's disease and other dementias. The main hope at the moment lies in a group of drugs called cholinesterase inhibitors or anticholinesterase drugs, which reduce the breakdown of acetylcholine, a chemical found in the brain. (See the answer to the next question for more details about how these drugs work).

Some examples of cholinesterase inhibitors are tacrine (also called Cognex), donepezil (Aricept) and rivastigmine (Exelon). Several studies have shown that these drugs appear to relieve some of the symptoms of Alzheimer's disease in some people, but that this effect wears off after a while. They do not work in all patients and their effect is variable. At the moment it is not possible to predict which people will be helped by them.

Although research suggests that cholinesterase inhibitors may help to slow the progress of Alzheimer's disease, they cannot halt the disease altogether nor reverse any brain damage that has already taken place. It seems that they are more likely to help people in the early stage of Alzheimer's disease. They are not expected to help people who already have severe dementia.

Only two cholinesterase inhibitors are currently available in the UK: donepezil and rivastigmine. These drugs appear to have few side effects. Other cholinesterase inhibitors will become available in the near future. Other compounds, which work in different ways, are also being developed and may become available in due course. (See p. 173 for more information.)

How do the new drugs for treating dementia work?

To date, the most promising new drugs belong to a group of drugs called cholinesterase inhibitors or anticholinesterase drugs. Drugs of this type work by reducing the breakdown of acetylcholine in the brain.

Acetylcholine is a chemical substance that occurs naturally in the brain, where it is continually being made and broken down. Acetylcholine is a 'neurotransmitter' – a chemical that enables nerve cells in the brain to pass messages to each other. In a normal brain, the total level of acetylcholine remains fairly constant. Research has shown, however, that the brains of many people with Alzheimer's disease have a reduced amount of acetylcholine, and it is thought that the loss of this chemical may result in deterioration of memory.

Much of the research so far carried out into finding ways of correcting acetylcholine deficiency in the brains of people with Alzheimer's disease has been directed towards increasing the amount of acetylcholine. However, the evidence seems to suggest that giving people this chemical directly does not help. The alternative approach of reducing the rate at which acetylcholine is broken down currently seems more promising, and has resulted in the development of the new cholinesterase-inhibiting drugs. (See the previous answer for more information on cholinesterase inhibitors.)

Why does the same drug have different names?

Most drugs have two names: a generic name and a brand name. The generic name is the official medical name for the basic active substance (e.g., donepezil) and is chosen by the British Pharmacopoeia Commission. The brand name (e.g., Aricept) is a name selected by the company that produces the drug. Different manufacturers give different names to the same generic drug in order to differentiate their product.

Are cholinesterase inhibitors, such as donepezil and rivastigmine, effective for all people with Alzheimer's disease?

Anticholinesterase drugs seem to help some, but by no means all, people with Alzheimer's disease. Even when they are effective, they go only some way towards reducing memory problems. In many people, there is only minimal benefit or none at all. Unfortunately, it is not possible to tell in advance who will respond well to this type of treatment. The effectiveness of the drug is not affected by a taker's age, sex or ethnic origin.

Do anticholinesterase drugs have any side effects?

Any type of drug may cause side effects and sometimes these are unpredictable. Anticholinesterase drugs are relatively new and not all their side effects may yet be apparent. However, the more recent anticholinesterase drugs appear to have few side effects, although some people may experience nausea and vomiting, diarrhoea and sleepiness. Side effects vary from drug to drug and from person to person but tend to become less troublesome after a few weeks.

My aunt recently started on donepezil and seems a little better. How long can I expect this effect to last?

A response to donepezil is frequently seen within the first few weeks of starting the drug. However, it is likely that this response will not last for more than a few months or a year. A further problem may be that once people stop taking the drug, their memory may deteriorate more rapidly, so that they may soon find themselves in the position they would have been in if they had never taken the drug at all.

Treating symptoms

My husband, who has Alzheimer's disease, sleeps very little and is very restless at night. This disturbs my sleep too and I am getting very tired. Could he take sleeping pills, or might they make him more confused?

The decision to give sleeping pills to someone with Alzheimer's disease should not be taken lightly. Doctors generally agree that sedatives, such as sleeping pills and tranquillisers, can increase confusion. They can also cause unsteadiness of gait, which may lead to falls. It is therefore wise to avoid them if at all possible.

Possible alternatives to sleeping pills may include practical measures, such as providing plenty of activity during the day (see Chapter 5 for ideas), avoiding too many cat-naps, avoiding caffeine, not giving a heavy meal late at night, giving a relaxing bath before bed and making sure that the bedroom is warm and comfortable.

In some circumstances, however, the use of sleeping pills or tranquillisers is necessary. They may be needed, for example, if the affected person's wakefulness is preventing the only carer from getting a proper night's sleep, causing long-term tiredness and making it difficult to cope during the day. Another reason for a doctor to prescribe a sedative is if the person with Alzheimer's disease is at risk from night-time wandering and confusion.

You say that you are getting very tired. In view of this, it would probably be sensible talk to your doctor about the possibility of sleeping pills for your husband, at least for a time.

My mother's dementia seems to be getting worse and she often becomes very agitated and upset. I used to be able to distract or calm her myself, but she no longer responds to my efforts. Might drugs help?

In general, doctors will try to avoid using drugs to treat anxiety and agitation in people with Alzheimer's disease. Drugs, such as tranquillisers, can have side effects that outweigh their benefits.

Careful management of a person with Alzheimer's disease and plenty of reassurance if he or she is starting to become upset can often work wonders, at least in the early stages of the disease. However, as in your mother's case, management can become more difficult as the disease progresses.

Your mother's doctor may be able to help her without resorting to tranquillisers. For example, a physical examination may reveal that your mother's increased agitation is due to a treatable pain, perhaps from constipation (see the next answer for more on this). Another possibility might be for your mother's doctor to involve a clinical psychologist who has experience of working with people with Alzheimer's disease. He or she may be able to offer you useful advice on how to carry on managing your mother.

However, in some cases, especially in the later stages of Alzheimer's disease or if a person is suffering from long-term anxiety disorder, drugs may be the best option for increasing the quality of life for sufferers and carers alike. (Also see below for more information on the advantages and disadvantages of using tranquillisers.)

I understand that constipation can cause increased agitation in people with Alzheimer's disease. Might laxative drugs be useful?

It is true that constipation can cause increased agitation in people with Alzheimer's disease. In the first instance, constipation is best treated by dietary measures. More bran, fruit and vegetables will often help to ease the problem. Some people may find such foods difficult to accept, but others seem to thrive on them. Taking plenty to drink during the day, and regular exercise when possible, should also help.

It is recognised, however, that further treatment is needed in some cases. A doctor will be able to give advice on the possible use of laxatives, such as Regulan, Fybogel and lactulose. In some cases, where poor coordination and weak anal sphincter muscles are factors, a regular enema may be the best treatment.

I've heard that giving tranquillisers can make people with Alzheimer's disease worse. Is this true?

There is always a risk when taking any sort of medication

but this should be balanced in each case against the potential benefits. Tranquillisers are no exception.

The point of giving tranquillisers is to calm someone down if they are agitated, or to give them a restful night's sleep if they would otherwise be up and about disturbing not only themselves but also carers and other family members.

The main disadvantages of tranquillisers are that they can make people sleepy and more confused during the day. They can also reduce coordination, causing falls. This is particularly a problem in older people, who may not be able to get up easily off the floor, even with the help of a carer. Furthermore, older people with brittle bones may sustain a fracture if they fall. For these reasons it is always important to make sure that the dose of tranquilliser is correct: not too little so that it doesn't work and not too much so that it makes people drowsy or uncoordinated. If you are worried about someone you care for being given tranquillisers you should talk to his or her doctor.

Some tranquillising medication (known as antipsychotic drugs or neuroleptic drugs) may occasionally cause side effects that make people more restless rather than less. If someone starts taking these tablets and seems more restless as a result, you should let the doctor know in case the dose can be reduced or the tablets stopped altogether.

Our doctor has prescribed temazepam to help my husband sleep. I gather this medicine is similar to Valium. Is it addictive?

Temazepam and diazepam (Valium) are commonly used tranquillisers that can be very useful for calming people who are agitated and helping them to get to sleep. Tranquillisers of this type may cause dependence (a form of addiction) in some people. This means that it can be difficult to stop these tablets, and doing so may cause withdrawal symptoms, notably feeling unwell or anxious.

Addiction is only usually a problem if these drugs are taken for three weeks or more. If you are worried about your husband becoming addicted, talk to your doctor. Sometimes the risks of addiction are outweighed by the benefits of the medication. Alternatively, there are other medicines that help sleep that are possibly less addictive. Sometimes, general measures, such as avoiding caffeine and having a relaxing bath before bed, may be enough.

Other medicines your doctor may prescribe, including drugs known as neuroleptics (or antipsychotics) and anti-depressants, are not addictive. Don't be afraid to discuss with the doctor any medications that are prescribed.

My wife, who has Alzheimer's, seems to be suffering from hallucinations, which sometimes make her very distressed. Can anything be done to help?

Hallucinations – in which a person sees, hears, smells or feels something when there is nothing there to cause it – are fairly common in people with Alzheimer's disease. However, the tendency to suffer from them varies, not only from day to day but also over time. Sometimes, hallucinations, especially visual hallucinations, are worse at night or in poor lighting, when patients are more apt to misinterpret what they see. If someone becomes more agitated at night, then the occurrence of hallucinations should be considered as a possibility. In many people, hallucinations seem to stop occurring as the disease progresses.

Treatment of hallucinations in a person with Alzheimer's disease should begin with trying to reassure the sufferer that what they are experiencing is not really happening. However, many people will not accept this reassurance and, as a result, doctors may have to resort to medication. Medication can help to reduce hallucinations. The mainstay of treatment is the use of antipsychotic drugs. Small doses of these drugs may result in a substantial reduction in the hallucinations. However, your wife's doctor will need to weigh up carefully the potential benefit of giving these drugs to your wife against their potential side effects, which include worsening confusion.

**Is there any point in treating other mental health
conditions, such as depression and anxiety, in someone
who has been diagnosed with Alzheimer's disease?**

During the course of a dementia such as Alzheimer's disease,
treatment may be needed for a variety of physical and
mental disorders.

It is very important always to obtain appropriate treatment for physical illnesses when someone has Alzheimer's
disease, since quite minor disorders can produce either
worsening of the dementia, or acute confusion. Many underlying medical illnesses can be treated.

Of the recognised mental illnesses, depression and anxiety
are those most likely to be experienced by people with
dementia. Depression is relatively common in elderly people.
Some people with Alzheimer's disease will have suffered
recurring bouts of depression before developing the dementia.
Others will be suffering from a depressive illness for the first
time. Given that depression can lead to failure to eat and
drink, causing severe weight loss, unexplained behaviour
problems and sheer misery, it certainly merits treatment.
(See the next answer for more information.)

Anxiety frequently accompanies the early stages of a
dementia and, at this stage, is usually best dealt with by
reassurance rather than drug therapy. Later, when reassurance is more difficult, and in people who suffer from long-term
anxiety disorder, medication can be useful.

**How do you treat someone who has depression and
dementia?**

The two mainstays of treatment for depression are medication
and talking therapies (psychotherapy and cognitive therapy).
Both may sometimes have a role in the treatment of depression in a person with dementia.

In someone with quite an advanced dementia, however,
talking therapies are not usually possible because the person
is too confused and cannot concentrate for long enough.

Furthermore, these treatments are sometimes not easily obtainable and can be expensive. For these reasons, many doctors resort to medication in the first instance.

There are several different types of antidepressant tablets. Some of the older antidepressants are possibly best avoided because they may cause side effects that make memory problems worse. Some newer antidepressants, such as those belonging to the group known as serotonin specific reuptake inhibitors, do not have these side effects.

It is often difficult to be sure whether someone with a dementia such as Alzheimer's disease is also suffering from depression. In view of this, a doctor may decide to prescribe a course of antidepressant tablets and then see what happens. The tablets will have to be taken regularly for at least two weeks before there is any obvious effect. The signs of an improvement can be quite subtle, perhaps just less agitation and a more cheerful disposition. In some cases, there are also improvements in memory. It is important, however, not to be too optimistic about any such improvements in memory. The dementia itself does not respond to treatment with antidepressant drugs.

Surgery

We have been told that my husband has Alzheimer's disease. Would an operation on his brain help?

At present there is no operation that can help people with Alzheimer's disease. On the contrary, there is a risk that any type of operation will make a person with Alzheimer's disease more confused.

Research is currently being performed into the possibility of transplanting brain cells into the brains of people with Alzheimer's disease, as has been tried as a treatment for some people with Parkinson's disease. However, this research is at a very early stage and it may not lead to an operation of this type ever becoming widely available. (See p. 174 for more details.)

One very rare form of dementia, called normal pressure hydrocephalus (see p. 25), may possibly be helped by an operation to drain fluid from the brain. Diagnosis of normal pressure hydrocephalus can be difficult, but it is extremely unlikely that your husband has this condition rather than Alzheimer's disease. Also, even if someone does have normal pressure hydrocephalus, an operation is not always advised

My husband, who has recently been diagnosed as suffering from Alzheimer's disease, has finally been offered a long-awaited hip-replacement operation. Should he have the operation or might it make his confusion worse?

As a general rule, the medical and surgical needs of patients with Alzheimer's disease are the same as those of unaffected elderly people. Sufferers from Alzheimer's disease are entitled to appropriate treatment for physical illnesses, and this sometimes includes operations.

Removal of a person with Alzheimer's disease from home to hospital surroundings, and the use of anaesthetic and even pain-relieving drugs, may temporarily increase confusion. There is also a small risk of permanent mental deterioration. This risk of increased confusion is generally considered acceptable in life-threatening situations, or in the case of an operation that will improve a patient's quality of life.

There are, however, particular problems in the case of a hip-replacement operation. The success of this operation depends on the patient's ability to understand and co-operate with a rehabilitation programme. The rate at which older people in general, and people with dementias such as Alzheimer's disease in particular, can progress is often too slow for an ordinary orthopaedic ward. In some hospitals the geriatric department runs a recovery ward in conjunction with the orthopaedic team. Difficulties occur when the orthopaedic staff are unaware of a patient's mental state.

Whether or not it is a good idea for your husband to have his hip-replacement operation will depend on the details of his particular case. In view of this, your best action would be to discuss the situation with the orthopaedic staff at the hospital in consultation with the local geriatric or psycho-geriatric service, so that a proper assessment of risks and benefits can be made.

Psychological treatments

What is involved in reminiscence therapy? And is it useful for people with dementia?

Reminiscence therapy involves stimulating the recollection of events or memories from the past. This is achieved by using music, videotapes or pictures (for example, films of trams or photographs of early cinema idols) or by providing articles such as food packaging or items of clothing from past eras. Reminiscence therapy is usually carried out in small groups. Items to help stimulate memories are available from Age Concern and the Alzheimer's Disease Society (addresses in Appendix 1).

People with dementia often appear to enjoy reminiscence therapy, although it probably does not prevent the memory getting worse in the long run.

Can you explain what reality orientation is? Does it do any good?

Reality orientation is a technique in which people caring for individuals with dementia take every opportunity to orien-tate people with dementia. For example, a member of staff in a hospital or nursing home may remind someone with dementia where they are and what time of day it is each time they meet. Staff members would also disagree whenever someone with dementia says something that is incorrect.

Reality orientation is a controversial technique and is not practised everywhere. Some authorities believe it improves orientation and awareness of the surroundings, whereas others have criticised it for being ineffective and insensitive.

I am in charge of a nursing home and some of my residents disturb the others by shouting and screaming. I am aware of research criticising the over-use of drugs in nursing homes. Are there any other ways I can tackle this problem?

Sometimes people with dementia shout or scream because they are in pain or discomfort due to various causes (such as those given as causes of restlessness on p. 88). When no cause can be identified, it may be possible to stop difficult behaviour without resort to drugs.

If the behaviour is precipitated by a particular event or situation, it may be possible to take action to avoid it. For example, if shouting occurs when someone is waiting for a meal, making sure that they are given their meal first may sometimes improve matters. If there is no obvious trigger, it may help to give the person with dementia more attention when they are not shouting or screaming rather than responding to them immediately they start to shout or scream. This has the effect of rewarding the more desirable behaviour rather than reinforcing the difficult behaviour.

Our local hospital is raising money for a Snoezelen. What is this?

Snoezelens have now been installed in a number of hospitals, care homes and day centres. A Snoezelen is a special room designed to gently stimulate the senses while also helping agitated people to relax. There are comfortable places to sit, coloured moving lights and restful music. Some Snoezelens also have pleasant aromas. Although more research is needed into the value of this form of therapy, Snoezelens are thought to be useful for some people with dementia.

Complementary medicine

Might alternative or complementary medicine help someone with Alzheimer's disease?

There is no reason why a person with Alzheimer's disease should not try alternative or complementary therapies. There are many possible approaches, including homeopathy, acupuncture, massage, aromatherapy and spiritual healing. Unfortunately, because of the nature of these treatments, they are often 'unproven', but this should not stop you from seeking advice or trying them out. One note of caution: if you do decide to try a form of alternative or complementary therapy, it is always wise to consult a practitioner who is accredited by a professional body. Further information is available from the Institute for Complementary Medicine (address in Appendix 1).

My wife has been diagnosed with Alzheimer's disease and I'd like her to see a spiritual healer. How do we go about this?

Spiritual healers, also known as contact healers or faith healers, see people suffering from a wide variety of illnesses, including Alzheimer's disease. As with other complementary treatments, you would be wise to consult a practitioner who is bound by the professional code of conduct of a recognised organisation. There are several organisations of spiritual healers in the United Kingdom. Further information may be obtained from the Institute for Complementary Medicine or The National Federation of Spiritual Healers (addresses in Appendix 1).

13
Research

Introduction

Worldwide, there is an enormous amount of research into Alzheimer's disease and other dementias. The need for research is urgent because people are living longer, and the number of people suffering from dementias is increasing. Dementia is a distressing illness and its effects are far-reaching. The need to care for people with dementia takes a toll both on individuals doing the caring and on governments

169

providing the resources. This chapter has questions on the major areas of research and on various research-related issues.

Research overview

What are the main areas of research into dementia at at the present time?

The three main areas of research at the present time are: looking for the causes of dementia; developing drugs that can slow down the progression of dementia; and trying to find better ways of helping carers.

Much has already been discovered about the changes that take place in the brains of people with various types of dementia. However, much less is known about why these changes occur. Until researchers can find the underlying causes of Alzheimer's disease and other dementias, there is little hope for finding a cure.

Research into treatments for dementia continues to concentrate on developing drugs that can slow down the progression of the disease. Some drugs, for example cholinesterase-inhibiting drugs (see p. 156), seem to work for some people, at least for a few months. However, much more research is still needed to improve these and other possible drug treatments.

Important research is also being carried out to try and identify the best ways of helping carers to cope with the enormous difficulties they face (see p. 181).

Where can I get up-to-date, accurate information on research into Alzheimer's Disease?

Information on research into Alzheimer's disease is available from the Alzheimer's Disease Society and from Alzheimer Scotland (addresses in Appendix 1). These organisations both try to keep abreast of new research developments in the

United Kingdom and elsewhere, and both frequently produce easy-to-understand information sheets on new developments. The Alzheimer's Disease Society's monthly newsletter also provides research information. Each month, a researcher contributes an article on an up-to-date research topic.

Newspapers, magazines, radio and television programmes quite often give coverage to research into Alzheimer's disease and other dementias. However, it is important to remember that not all the information they give is accurate. Also, there is a tendency for the popular press to make too much of apparently promising early research findings. All too often, the claims turn out to have been exaggerated or misplaced.

If you have access to the Internet, you may find this is a useful source of information on Alzheimer's disease research.

Where does the funding for medical research into diseases such as Alzheimer's disease come from?

There are three main sources of funding for medical research. These are: the government (using revenue from taxation), pharmaceutical companies and charities.

In the United Kingdom, the government's contribution to medical research funding takes different forms. It includes money allocated to the National Health Service (NHS), the Medical Research Council (MRC), the Department of Health and also the universities (through the Department for Education and Employment). Government money finances most of the long-term infrastructure for medical research (including hospitals and university research departments), as well as providing money for specific medical research projects.

Pharmaceutical companies together contribute the largest share (in excess of 50%) of all medical research funding in the United Kingdom. Developing new drugs costs a great deal of money, but the profits from a successful drug for a common disease such as Alzheimer's disease are potentially enormous. Pharmaceutical companies fund research in their own laboratories and also often run drug trials (see p. 176) involving many researchers in centres around the country.

Charities, such as the Alzheimer's Disease Society, also spend significant amounts of money on research each year. Charity money is generally spent on financing specific research projects, which are carefully selected for quality and effectiveness. In recent years, the Alzheimer's Disease Society has funded research into diagnosis, brain injury, preventing falls, carers' stress and the neurochemistry of Alzheimer's disease.

Is there international collaboration of research into Alzheimer's disease as there is with AIDS?

Specific research projects into dementias tend to be locally or nationally based. However, the researchers involved in these projects belong to a wider scientific community. Scientists from many countries often come together at international conferences to share their ideas and present their research findings. Among the groups that organise such conferences are the International Psychogeriatric Association and Alzheimer's Disease International. Researchers also read medical journals published in other countries, and communicate with colleagues in other countries via the Internet.

Despite a lot of media hype, it seems to me that not many new treatments for Alzheimer's disease ever see the light of day. Why is this?

Thousands of scientists around the world are working hard to find better treatments for dementia. When potentially good treatments are found, this is exciting news and they receive a lot of publicity in the media. However, many 'discoveries' are never heard of again, either because they don't work as well as was initially thought or because they are found to be unsafe. Even when a line of research does lead to a new treatment – such as the drug donepezil (see p. 156) – there will always have been a research period of several years between the initial research findings and the granting of a license to make the drug available for use.

What guarantee is there that research findings that suggest that a new Alzheimer's treatment may be effective will ever be followed up?

Although there is no guarantee, it is almost certain that any new treatments that might to be effective in treating Alzheimer's disease will be followed up. There is currently a lot of interest in finding treatments that will reduce the misery and economic burden that Alzheimer's disease brings to its sufferers and their carers. Charities concerned with Alzheimer's disease, government and also pharmaceutical companies are all very interested in this area of research.

Experimental treatments

I have read about donepezil for treating Alzheimer's disease. Are any other drugs being developed?

Donepezil belongs to a group of drugs called cholinesterase inhibitors (see p. 156). Rivastigmine, another cholinesterase inhibitor, is also available. Other drugs of this type, including metrifonate and galanthamine, are expected to become available in the near future.

Many other drugs are being investigated. These include drugs that directly increase the amount of acetylcholine (see p. 156) in the brain, and also drugs that protect the brain from damage, such as vitamin E and selegiline (used in the treatment of Parkinson's disease). Oestrogen and aspirin may also prove useful. Moss and plant extracts, including Gingko biloba, are also being investigated.

What is nerve growth factor? I have heard that this may be useful in treating Alzheimer's disease.

One type of brain cell, known as cholinergic neurones, die off as Alzheimer's disease progresses. These cells produce the chemical known as acetylcholine, which seems to be involved in the working of memory. As the cholinergic neurones die off, the level of acetylcholine in the brain falls, and the memory gets worse. Nerve growth factor is a compound that stimulates these cells, possibly slowing the rate of death.

Scientists in Sweden have recently infused nerve growth factor into a person with Alzheimer's disease and the results look promising. However, much more work needs to be done before this treatment becomes generally available. The nerve growth factor was injected directly into the brain, which makes this treatment both difficult and dangerous.

I'm sure I have read that doctors can transplant brain tissue to cure Alzheimer's disease, like they have done with Parkinson's disease. Is this the case?

Not yet. The idea of transplanting brain tissue to treat Alzheimer's disease is still in its infancy. Also, even if research shows that such treatment will work, it is unlikely to be widely available for many years.

The idea of a transplant is based on the discovery that brain cells of a particular type – called cholinergic neurones – die off as Alzheimer's disease progresses. These neurones produce the chemical acetylcholine, which seems to play a part in memory. If cholinergic neurones could be transplanted into the brain of someone with Alzheimer's disease, then it is possible that memory might be improved. A similar approach, using a different type of cell, has been tried, with limited success, in the treatment of Parkinson's disease.

Helping with research

My husband has been told he's got dementia but that it is in quite an early stage. I have talked this through with him and we are keen to help research into a cure. What can be done?

Quite a number of studies are currently being conducted into new treatments for dementia. To take part in a study, your husband will need to meet various entry criteria. This usually means: that there must be no doubt about the diagnosis of dementia; that the dementia is not at an advanced stage; and that the person is otherwise medically quite fit.

It is probably worth talking first to your husband's GP. He or she may be able to put you in contact with a doctor (probably a psychiatrist, geriatrician or neurologist) at the local hospital, who may have information about studies being conducted near you. Alternatively, the Alzheimer's Disease Society or Alzheimer Scotland (see Appendix 1) may have information about trials being conducted in your area.

My wife has Alzheimer's disease and I am keen to see that something good comes out of this. On her death, I'd like her brain to be donated for medical research. But is this possible without her consent? She is now too ill to give that consent herself.

It is possible for your wife's brain to be used for medical research without her consent. Whether or not you should suggest this course depends to a great extent on what you think your wife would have wanted. If you know, for example, that she was against organ donation or research, then you probably should not allow the brain to be used for research. However, if you feel that it would have been her wish to help in medical research in this way, then arrangements can be made for her brain to be donated after death.

I have heard there is a brain bank for the brains of people who have died of Alzheimer's disease. What can researchers learn from these donated brains?

Scientists in many countries, including the UK and the USA, run brain banks, where the brains of people who died of Alzheimer's disease and other dementias are stored and studied. Looking at the brains of people who have died of dementia can provide a great deal of information to scientists searching for the causes and cures of dementia.

One reason why it is so useful to examine the brain of a dementia sufferer after death is that it can be very difficult when somebody is alive to be absolutely certain of the type of dementia they are suffering from. Only by using a micro-scope to study removed brain tissue after a person's death is it usually possible to make a definite diagnosis.

It can also be useful for researchers to be able to study the brain of someone who has died with dementia in conjunc-tion with other research carried out when the person was still alive. This is useful, for example, when investigating the causes of dementia and also when trying to assess the effects of experimental treatments.

Drug trials

What processes must a drug go through before it becomes available for general use?

Before any drug can be made generally available, either on prescription or over the counter, it has to undergo numerous tests to make sure that it works and also that it is safe. Only a tiny proportion of the drugs that are under development ever become available for use by patients.

If a drug is thought to be of potential use, it is first of all tested in the laboratory and then its safety tested on healthy human volunteers. Following this, the drug may be given to selected patients taking part in carefully monitored drug trials. If extensive testing shows that a drug is both useful and safe, it may be be approved in the UK by the Committee on Safety of Medicines (CSM). This may take many years from the first discovery of the drug. Only after the CSM has approved and licensed a drug for use in the UK, can a pharmaceutical company market it, or doctors prescribe it to patients other than those taking part in drug trials.

What happens if we agree that my husband will help in a drug trial?

Drug trials are usually conducted at many sites throughout the country, so it should not be necessary to travel very far to take part. The usual procedure would be for you and your husband to go and see a doctor or other researcher involved with the trial. You will both probably be interviewed and asked to fill in a questionnaire. Your husband will then probably be given a thorough physical examination, a memory test, blood tests and perhaps a test of heart function.

If your husband is considered eligible for the trial, he will be given a supply of tablets. These may be either the new medication, or a placebo (an inactive compound, usually a harmless sugar). Neither you, your husband nor the researchers you see will know which tablets he receives. You will be given instructions about how many tablets your husband needs to take, and how often. It is important that you try to make sure that these instructions are followed.

You and your husband will then need to see the researcher regularly, usually for a period of at least 16 weeks, so that your husband's condition can be monitored. Your husband will probably need to have further blood tests and memory tests each time you see the researcher. You may be asked about how you think your husband is doing.

My husband is taking part in a study that is testing a new treatment for Alzheimer's disease. But I have not been told whether he is having the proper drug or the placebo. Why is this?

Your husband is in what is known as a placebo-controlled trial. In such trials, some of the participants are given the active drug, while others are given a placebo (an inactive compound, usually a harmless sugar) that looks exactly the same. Participants are not told whether they are being given the active drug or the placebo, because giving people this information can affect the results of the trial. The trial will also be what is called a double-blind trial, meaning that the researchers you see will also not know which is which, because this knowledge might affect how they treat different participants and so also affect the results of the trial.

The reason for giving some people a placebo when a new medication is under trial is that the actual participation in a trial can in itself lead to an improvement which may mistakenly be thought to be due to the drug. For example, regular visits to the hospital, completing questionnaires and chatting with a researcher may in itself make some people seem brighter and less confused. Therefore, people involved in this sort of trial are treated in exactly the same way whether they are getting the active drug or the placebo. If neither you, your husband nor the researcher knows whether your husband is on the placebo or the active drug, then any changes that are picked up in the people receiving the active drug are likely to be due to the drug itself rather than to the effect of being in a trial.

At the end of the trial, when the results are looked at, the overall response of all those who took the placebo is compared with the response of those taking the active drug. If there is an improvement in the group that took the active drug, compared with the placebo group, then this suggests that the new drug works. Also, even if both groups get worse, but the group on the active drug becomes less unwell than the placebo group, then this suggests that the active drug is still of some benefit. The new medication may be slowing down the progress of the illness. Without a placebo group as a control, this benefit would be missed by the trial.

My husband has been on a trial of a new drug and seems to be doing well. The trial has now stopped, can he continue the drug?

To a great extent, the answer depends on the company that is conducting the trial. In some instances, patients who have done well with a particular drug will be able to continue taking it. In other instances, this will not be possible, at least for the time being. If the trial proves successful, then your husband's doctor would, of course, be able to prescribe the drug to your husband when it becomes generally available.

When people are in a drug trial, why do they have to make so many visits to the hospital? Why not just see them once at the end?

Frequent hospital visits to see the people running the trial may seem time-consuming but they are important. What researchers are looking for in a trial is a trend to an improvement. If a participant's memory was tested only at the beginning and end of a trial, then the researchers would not know whether the participant was simply having a better or a worse day when followed up. Another important reason for frequent visits during the course of a trial is that this allows the researchers to monitor trial participants in case they develop side effects that may mean that they should stop taking the drug.

What happens if the drug given in a trial turns out to be harmful?

Before any new drug is given to patients, even in a trial, it will have been tested very thoroughly. It will have been subjected to laboratory tests, and then given to a group of healthy volunteers. After this, it will be given to a small number of patients in a very closely monitored preliminary trial. Only after a drug has passed all these tests, will it be considered for a more general drug trial.

Despite all the precautions taken during testing, some drugs do turn out to have rare side effects that only become obvious after these drugs have been given to large numbers of people. There is a small risk in taking any drug, but the risk may be slightly higher with new drugs. For this reason, researchers conducting a drug trial will keep a very close eye on all trial participants and will want to hear straight away if any worrying side effects appear.

Sometimes, a drug does produce unpredictable side effects. If this happens, and someone suffers as a result, then they may be eligible for compensation in some circumstances.

Other areas of research

What can genetic research tell us about the development of Alzheimer's disease, and how might this information be put to practical use?

Genetic research has already identified several genes that play a part in the development of Alzheimer's disease (see p. 6). It is hoped that further research will be able to show how abnormal genes actually cause or assist the disease to develop.

The first practical application of genetic research into the causes of Alzheimer's disease has been the development of a screening test (see p. 39) for the rare inherited form of the disease. The usefulness of possibly developing genetic tests for other forms of Alzheimer's disease seems less clear at present, especially in the absence of a cure for the disease.

In theory, it might be possible at some stage to replace or repair damaged genes, including those implicated in the development of Alzheimer's disease. However, research of this type is still very much in its infancy and practical results cannot be expected for many years yet.

Has any research been carried out into non-medical treatments for dementia?

There has been a certain amount of research into various non-medical treatments for dementia. For example, researchers have looked into the use of bright lights and music to help with agitated behaviour, the use of strong magnetic fields to try and improve memory, and the effects on the brain of physical and mental exercise. Some of the findings look promising, but more research is needed.

Is there any research into ways of helping carers to cope with looking after people with dementia?

This is an important area of research. Most people with dementia are cared for in their own homes, which places a heavy burden on the family members who care for them. Research is concentrated on ways of lightening this burden. It has been shown, for example, that day care (see p. 116) significantly reduces the stress on carers. In addition, it has been demonstrated that it is an efficient use of hospital or care home beds to provide respite care (see p. 117) for people with dementia so that their carers can have a break.

Is there any research showing how carers can be helped to improve how they look after their relatives with dementia?

There has been a lot of research into how caring for someone with dementia affects the carer and how stress on the carer can be reduced. Research has shown that, on the whole, carers do an excellent job despite having no formal training. Many carers experience a major change in their own lifestyle as a result of caring for someone with dementia. Despite this, many carers tend not to make full use of the support that is available to them from other family members, Social Services and carers' support groups. The demands of caring for someone with dementia result in an increased risk of physical problems and depression in some carers. To some extent, these problems can be reduced by having help from other members of the family, learning how to cope with problem behaviours and having good support and information from doctors, nurses and other professionals.

One study in Australia showed that carers of people with dementia improved their quality of care if they were given an intensive training course at the day centre attended by the person they were caring for. These carers also seemed to be less stressed by the demands made on them.

Glossary

Terms appearing in *italics* in these definitions refer to other entries in the glossary.

acetylcholine One of a group of chemicals known as *neurotransmitters*. Found throughout the brain, acetylcholine enables nerve cells to communicate with each other. In *Alzheimer's disease*, the levels of acetylcholine are lower than usual.

acute confusional state A condition in which a person becomes confused over a matter of hours or days. Possible causes include infections in the chest or bladder, a *stroke*, various medicines and even constipation. It usually gets better if the cause is treated.

AIDS Abbreviation for Acquired Immune Deficiency Syndrome.

Alzheimer's disease The commonest cause of *dementia*. It usually begins after the age of 65 and results in gradual, progressive loss of memory and other functions of the brain.

amyloid A protein that is found in the brains of people with *Alzheimer's disease*. It is deposited throughout the brain in microscopic clumps known as plaques. Its function is unknown and it may be the cause of the deterioration of brain function.

anticholinergic drugs A term for drugs that reverse or inhibit the action of *acetylcholine* on nerve cells.

anticholinesterase drugs A group of drugs, also known as cholinesterase inhibitors, that stop the breakdown of *acetylcholine*. These drugs may help to slow down the progression of *Alzheimer's disease* in some people. *Donepezil* (Aricept) is an example.

antipsychotic drugs A range of *tranquillisers*, also known as neuroleptic drugs, that help to reduce symptoms of aggression.

182

They may also be used for treating *hallucinations*. Examples include chlorpromazine (Largactil) and thioridazine (Melleril).

Aricept The brand name for *donepezil*.

brain bank The name used for a store of brains removed after death. Tissue taken from the brains of people who have died of *dementia* can provide invaluable material for research scientists looking for causes and a cure for the disease.

brain scan A general term to mean any investigation that produces pictures of the brain. A *CT scan* or *MRI scan* shows slices through the brain. A *SPECT scan* shows the brain's blood supply.

care manager A person from a *Social Services* department (or sometimes from *Community Health Services*) whose job it is to put together, monitor and review the care plan agreed after a *needs assessment* for *community care*.

carer In the broadest sense, a carer is a person who provides help and support to another person, usually a relative or friend. More specifically, a carer is someone who looks after another person who needs help with daily living and who would not otherwise be able to live independently at home.

CAT scan Abbreviation for Computerised Axial Tomography scan. Another name for a *CT scan*.

cerebral An adjective referring to the brain.

cerebral cortex The outer layers of the brain, involved in thinking, memory and the interpretation of perception or the senses.

cholinergic Referring to *acetylcholine*. For example, a cholinergic neurone is a brain cell that contains the chemical acetylcholine.

cholinesterase inhibitor An alternative name for an *anticholinesterase drug*.

chromosomes Microscopic thread-like structures that are present in all cells. They are collections of *genes*, which contain the genetic information that is transmitted from generation to generation.

CJD (Creutzfeldt Jakob disease) A very rare form of *dementia* caused by an infectious agent called a *prion*. As well as loss of memory, CJD commonly causes muscle jerking, blindness and problems with walking. Death occurs within a year or so.

clinical trial An investigation involving patients that is designed to find out whether a new drug or other treatment is beneficial in treating a disease.

cognitive tests Tests that assess how well a person can think and how well his or her memory is working.

cognitive therapy A treatment that involves getting a person to think differently about a problem or situation.

community care A term covering health and social care services delivered to people in the community, usually in their own home.

Community Health Council (CHC) A body that monitors the delivery of local health care. This body will take up complaints with the local hospital or GP on behalf of patients. CHCs also act as a link between patients and the providers of health care.

Community Health Services or **Community Health Trusts** Parts of the NHS which provide health care in people's own homes or in local clinics and health centres.

community psychiatric nurse (CPN) A community-based nurse who is specially trained to look after the psychological needs of people living at home.

complementary medicine An approach to health care that explores alternatives to conventional treatments. Acupuncture, *homeopathy*, aromatherapy and spiritual healing are examples of complementary therapies.

confusion A state in which problems with memory and concentration impair the function of the mind.

consultant A doctor who usually works from a hospital and who has specialist knowledge about a particular field of medicine. Consultants involved in the care of people with dementia include *geriatricians, neurologists* and *psychiatrists*.

continuing care Long-term care provided by a hospital under the NHS. Continuing care of people with dementia has now been largely replaced by care in private homes paid for personally or by *Social Services*.

CT scan A computerised tomography scan. This is an X-ray scan that results in a series of pictures of 'slices' through the brain. Also known as a *CAT scan*.

day care The provision of day-time care in a *day centre*. Day care for people with dementia may involve practical help, such as with bathing, chiropody, etc., and also activities, such as *reminiscence therapy* and exercises.

day centre A facility, run by a Health Authority, Social Services or a voluntary organisation, that provides *day care* for people who are unable to look after themselves. People attend the centre during the day and return home in the evenings.

dehydration A state in which there is insufficient water in the body. It occurs when a person's fluid intake fails to balance fluid lost through sweating, vomiting or diarrhoea.

dementia A term used to describe impairment of brain function, involving memory, thinking and concentration. Dementia usually becomes progressively worse, eventually making it impossible for someone to cope with living without help. There are many causes of dementia, including *Alzheimer's disease, vascular dementia, Lewy body disease* and *Pick's disease.*

depression An illness in which the main symptoms are feeling low, tearfulness and loss of enjoyment. Depression can affect sleep, appetite, motivation and concentration. It is treatable.

diagnosis The process of identifying and naming a disease from a person's symptoms and signs. Getting a diagnosis may only involve talking with the doctor and having a physical examination. In other cases, special investigations may need to be done as well.

disinhibition Loss of the feelings of shame or embarrassment that normally help control a person's actions. Disinhibition results in inappropriate or improper behaviour.

disorientation A state in which someone loses their awareness of time and place. For example, they may fail to recall the date or even the year, and may not be able to say where they are.

donepezil Also known by the brand name Aricept, donepezil is an *anticholinesterase drug.* Donepezil may slow down the progression of *Alzheimer's disease* in some people.

double blind trial A type of clinical trial in which different groups of people are given either a new treatment, a *placebo* or an established treatment. Neither the people in the trial nor those assessing the responses know which treatment any individual is given. This is to make sure that any improvement in a person's condition is not due simply to taking part in the trial.

Enduring Power of Attorney (EPA) A legal document in which one person gives another the power to handle his or her financial affairs. An EPA can only be drawn up if the person handing over this power can understand what he or she is doing. The EPA comes into force only after it has been officially registered.

enema The introduction of a medicine directly into the rectum through the back passage. The most common reason for giving an enema is to relieve constipation.

epidemiology The study of the occurrence of disease within a population rather than in an individual. Epidemiology can help to identify the causes of a disease and to show whether particular groups of people are more likely to develop it.

frontal lobe dementia A *dementia* in which the disease process mainly affects the *frontal lobes* of the brain. Memory is affected less than in other dementias, but there may be major problems with loss of motivation and *disinhibition*.

frontal lobes Parts of the *cerebral cortex* situated at the front of the brain. This is the area of the brain that controls movement of the body. It is also involved in 'higher functions', such as planning ahead, problem solving and initiative.

generic drug A drug that is sold under its official medical name (its generic name) rather than under a patented brand name.

genes Material contained within the chromosomes. Genes carry the blueprint for the body: information that dictates how our bodies are built up, including the colour of our eyes and skin, how tall we are, our gender and many other details. Some genes have defects, or mutations, that cause disease.

geriatrician A doctor who specialises in the treatment of physical illnesses in older people.

hallucination A perception (hearing, seeing, smelling or feeling something) without an appropriate stimulus. For example, hearing voices when there is no one there. Hallucinations are quite common in people with *dementia*.

HIV Abbreviation for Human Immunodeficiency Virus.

home care The provision of home care-workers to help look after people in their own homes, usually arranged by *Social Services*. Home care-workers generally provide personal care, such as help with washing and dressing, preparing meals and other activities of daily life.

home help Usually a person who provides practical help, such as with shopping and cleaning. Most do not provide personal care.

homeopathy A branch of complementary medicine based on the principle that 'like can cure like'. A homeopath will prescribe very dilute amounts of substances which in larger quantities would cause the same symptoms as the illness being treated.

Huntington's disease Also sometimes called Huntington's chorea, a disease in which mental deterioration is accompanied by involuntary twitching and muscle spasms.

incontinence Involuntary or inappropriate passing of urine or faeces. Help is available from continence advisors.

laxative A medicine that treats constipation either by providing more fibre or by stimulating the bowel.

Lewy body disease A type of *dementia* in which abnormal collections of protein, known as Lewy bodies, occur in the brain. People with Lewy body disease typically show more variation in their mental abilities from day to day than is usual with other dementias.

memory The retention in the mind of information that may be recalled later.

Mental Health Act (1983) An act of parliament that governs the treatment and care of individuals incapacitated through mental illness. A section of the act allows a person to be compulsorily detained and treated. Different acts apply in Scotland and Ireland.

mentally incapacitated Being unable, through mental disorder, to take charge of financial and other affairs.

MRI scan Abbreviation for Magnetic Resonance Imaging scan. A type of brain scan that creates pictures using a powerful magnetic field rather than X-rays.

multi-disciplinary Referring to a team made up of professionals from different specialities, typically including doctors, nurses, *psychologists, social workers* and *occupational therapists.*

multi-infarct dementia Another name for *vascular dementia.*

needs assessment The process by which *Social Services* and health professionals assess the services that a person should be provided with under local *community care* provisions.

neuroleptic drugs Another name for *antipsychotic drugs.*

neurologist A doctor who specialises in the diagnosis, treatment and management of diseases of the nervous system.

neurone A nerve cell.

neurotransmitters A group of chemicals in the brain that enable nerve cells to communicate with each other. Groups of adjacent nerve cells tend to use the same neurotransmitter. Examples include *acetylcholine*, serotonin and dopamine.

nursing home A care home which offers 24-hour nursing care.

occupational therapist A person who can advise on ways of helping someone to maintain their skills and independence for as long as possible. They can also advise on aids in their home.

Parkinson's disease A chronic disease of the nervous system that is characterised by slowness of movements, a tremor and an expressionless face. Some affected people also develop *dementia.*

PET scan Abbreviation for Positron Emission Tomography scan. A sophisticated brain scan which is able to look at the brain in great detail. It is not generally available in clinical practice.

physiotherapist A person trained to perform physical treatments for joint and muscle problems.

Pick's disease A rare *dementia* which commonly affects younger people than *Alzheimer's disease*. It affects language and personality before there is any significant change in memory.

placebo The name given in *double-blind trials* to the non-active substance with which an active drug is being compared. It is a 'dummy' version of the drug, identical in appearance to the drug being tested.

psychiatrist A doctor who specialises in the diagnosis and treatment of mental illness.

psychogeriatrician A doctor who specialises in the diagnosis and treatment of mental illness in older people.

psychologist Someone with training in psychology, the study of behaviour. Clinical psychologists assess and treat people who have mental disorders.

psychotherapy A 'talking therapy' which can help people to understand their own feelings and therefore feel more confident to deal with them.

reality orientation A psychological treatment in which every opportunity is taken to make people with dementia aware of the time, where they are and the world around them.

receiver A person appointed to take responsibility for handling the financial affairs of a person with dementia when that person is no longer able to do this for him- or herself. The receiver may be a close relative, a friend, the local authority or a solicitor.

reminiscence therapy A treatment that aims to stimulate people's memories by means of old films, pictures, music, etc.

residential home Accommodation for people who are no longer able to manage everyday tasks or to maintain an independent home of their own, but who do not normally need nursing care.

respite care A facility or resource that allows *carers* to have a break. Respite care may be provided in a *residential home* or *nursing home,* in a person's own home or with another family.

sedative drugs Drugs used to reduce symptoms of anxiety and agitation and to help people sleep. Sedative drugs can increase confusion in people with dementia.

sheltered housing Units where people can live independently but where there is a warden on call who can offer a certain amount of supervision. Some support services may also be available.

side effects The unwanted 'extra' effects that occur in addition to the desired therapeutic effects of a drug. Most drugs have some side effects. These will vary from person to person and commonly disappear when the body becomes used to a particular drug.

Snoozelon A special room designed to gently stimulate the senses and to calm people who are agitated.

Social Services A local government department responsible for the non-medical welfare care of people in need. Social Services departments organise *needs assessments* for people with *dementia* and provide services under *community care* provisions.

social worker A professional who can offer advice on practical matters in connection with finances, *day care* and accommodation. A social worker will look at problems in the context of the family and the community. Some specialise in mental illness.

SPECT scan A Single Photon Emission Computed Tomography scan. A highly technical investigation similar to a *PET scan*.

stroke A result of a haemorrhage in the brain, or of a blood clot in an artery of the brain, leading to paralysis of part or all of one side of the body, or loss of speech, or loss of consciousness or death. The paralysis may be sudden or gradual in onset.

support group A group, also known as a self help group, that aims to provide mutual support for its members. A support group gives *carers* an opportunity to share their feelings, problems and information with other people undergoing similar experiences.

thyroid A gland in the neck that produces a chemical known as thyroid hormone. This hormone is essential to the workings of the body. Thyroid hormone deficiency is a rare cause of *dementia*.

tranquillisers Drugs used to help people who are very anxious. These drugs can cause increased confusion in people with *dementia*.

vascular dementia A type of *dementia* associated with problems affecting the circulation of blood to the brain, such as may result from a series of small *strokes*.

vitamins Chemical compounds essential to health that are found in many foods. Vitamin deficiency is a rare cause of *dementia*.

voluntary organisation Any organisation run on a not-for-profit basis. Many of the people who work for voluntary organisations do so without payment.

Appendix 1

Useful addresses

Age Concern England
Astral House
1268 London Road
London SW16 4ER
Tel: 0181 679 8000

Age Concern Scotland
113 Rose Street
Edinburgh
EH2 3DT
Tel: 0131 220 3345

Alzheimer Scotland – Action on
    Dementia
22 Drumsheugh Gardens
Edinburgh
EH3 7RN
Tel: 0131 243 1453
Freephone helpline: 0800 317817

Alzheimer's Disease
    International
45/46 Lower Marsh
London SE1 7RG
Tel: 0171 620 3011

Alzheimer's Disease Society
Gordon House
10 Greencoat Place
London SW1P 1PH
Tel: 0171 306 0606
Helpline (Mon-Fri, 8a.m.- 6p.m.):
0845 300 0336

Alzheimer's Disease Society
(Northern Ireland)
403 Lisburn Road
Belfast BT9 7EW
Tel: 01232 664100

Alzheimer's Disease Society
(Wales)
Tonna Hospital
Neath
West Glamorgan SA11 3LX
Tel: 01639 641938

Alzheimer Society of Ireland
43 Northumberland Avenue
Dun Laoghaire
Co Dublin, Ireland
Tel: 01 284 6616
        00 3531 284 6616 (from UK)

Association of Crossroads Care
  Attendants Schemes
10 Regent Place
Rugby
Warwickshire CV21 2PN
Tel: 01788 573653

Benefits Agency
  The address and telephone
  number of your local
  Benefits Agency will be in
  the Phone Book, and in
  Yellow Pages under
  Social Services.

Benefits Enquiry Line (BEL)
  for people with disabilities
Freephone: 0800 882 200 (for
  England, Wales & Scotland)
Freephone: 0800 220 674 (for
  Northern Ireland)

CANDID
(Counselling and Diagnosis in
  Dementia)
National Hospital for
  Neurology & Neurosurgery
Queen Square
London WC1N 3BG
Tel: 0171 837 3611

Carers Association of Ireland
St Mary's Community Centre
Richmond Hill
Dublin 6
Ireland
Tel: 01 497 4498
    00 3531 497 4498 (from UK)

Carers National Association
20-25 Glasshouse Yard
London EC1A 4JS
Tel: 0171 490 8818
Helpline: 0171 490 8898

Christian Council on Ageing
Caponscleugh House
Allerwash, Fourstones
Hexham
Northumberland NE47 5AB
Tel: 01434 674271

Citizens Advice Bureaux (CABx)
  The address and telephone
  number of your local CAB
  will be in the Phone Book,
  and in Yellow Pages under
  Counselling and Advice.

CJD Support Network
Alzheimer's Disease Society
Gordon House
10 Greencoat Place
London SW1P 1PH
Tel: 0171 306 0606

Community Health Council
  The address and telephone
  number of your local CHC
  will be in the Phone Book
  and in Yellow Pages.

Continence Foundation
2 Doughty Street
London WC1N 2PH
Tel: 0171 404 6875

Counsel and Care
Twyman House
16 Bonny Street
London NW1 9PG
Tel: 0171 485 1566

Court of Protection
  See entry on p. 193 for
  Public Trust Office.

CRUSE – Bereavement Care
Cruse House
126 Sheen Road
Richmond
Surrey TW9 1UR
Tel: 0181 940 4818
Cruse Bereavement line:
  0181 332 7227

Dementia Relief Trust
Pegasus House
37-43 Sackville Street
London W1X 2DL
Tel: 0171 333 8115

Disabled Living Foundation
380-384 Harrow Road
London W9 2HU
Tel 0171 289 6111

DVLA
(Driver & Vehicle Licensing
  Agency)
Drivers' Medical Unit
Longview Road
Morriston
Swansea SA99 1TU
Tel: 01792 783686

Elderly Accommodation Council
46A Chiswick High Road
London W4 1SZ
Tel: 0181 995 9320

Health Authority
  The address and telephone
  number of your local Health
  Authority will be in the
  Phone Book, and in Yellow
  Pages under Health
  Authorities and Services.

Huntington's Disease
  Association
108 Battersea High Street
London SW11 3HP
Tel: 0171 223 7000

Institute for Complementary
  Medicine
15 Tavern Quay
London SE16 1TX
Tel: 0171 237 5165

Jewish Care
221 Golders Green Road
London NW11 9DQ
Tel: 0181 458 3282

Law Centre
  The address and telephone
  number of your local Law
  Centre will be in the
  Phone Book, and in Yellow
  Pages under Legal Services.

MIND
Granta House
15-19 Broadway
Stratford
London E15 4BQ
Tel: 0181 519 2122

National Federation of
   Spiritual Healers
Old Manor Farm Studio
Church Street
Sunbury-on-Thames
Middlesex TW16 6RG
Tel: 01932 783164
Referrals only: 0189 161 6080

Parkinson's Disease Society
22 Upper Woburn Place
London WC1II 0RA
Tel: 0171 383 3513

Public Trust Office
Stewart House
24 Kingsway
London WC2B 6JX
Tel: 0171 664 7300

RADAR
   (Royal Association for
   Disability and Rehabilitation)
Unit 12, City Forum
250 City Road
London EC1V 8AF
Tel: 0171 250 3222

Relate
Herbert Gray College
Little Church Street
Rugby
Warwickshire CV21 3AP
Tel: 01788 573241 / 560811

Relatives Association
5 Tavistock Place
London WC1H 9SN
Tel: 0171 916 6055

Samaritans
National helpline: 0345 909090

Social Security
   The address and telephone
   number of your local office
   will be in the Phone Book
   under Benefits Agency,
   and in Yellow Pages under
   Social services.

Stroke Association
Stroke House
Whitecross Street
London EC1Y 8JJ
Tel: 0171 490 7999

Terrence Higgins Trust
52-54 Grays Inn Road
London WC1X 8JU
Tel: 0171 831 0330
Helpline: 0171 242 1010

United Kingdom Home Care
   Association
42B Banstead Road
Carshalton Beeches
Surrey SM5 3NW
Tel: 0181 288 1551

Winged Fellowship Trust
Angel House
20/32 Pentonville Road
London N1 9XD
Tel: 0171 833 2594

Appendix 2

Some other reading

Alzheimer's disease and dementia

Living with Alzheimer's Disease, by Dr. Gordon Wilcock, published by Penguin, 1990

Understanding dementia, by Alan Jacques, published by Churchill Livingstone, 2nd edition, 1992

Caring

Caring for the person with dementia, Bob Woods & Chris Lay, published by the Alzheimer's Disease Society, 1996

Coping with dementia: a handbook for carers, by Kate Fearnley & others, published by the Health Education Board for Scotland, 1996

Exchanging ideas: ideas, suggestions and helpful hints for carers of people with Alzheimer's disease, compiled by Ann Blofield, published by the Alzheimer's Disease Society, 1991

The 36 hour day: a family guide for caring at home, by Nancy L. Mace & others, published by Age Concern, 1993

Person to person, by Tom Kitwood & Kathleen Bredin, Gale Centre Publications, 2nd edition, 1992

Research

Opening the Mind: new frontiers in Alzheimer's research, published by the Alzheimer's Disease Society, 1996

Autobiography, biography and novels

Living in the Labyrinth, by Diana Friel McGowin, published by Mainsale Press, 1994

Caring for Maria, by Bernard Heywood, published by Element Books, 1994

Scar Tissue, by Michael Ignatieff, published by Chatto & Windus, 1993

Have the Men Had Enough?, by Margaret Forster, published by Chatto & Windus, 1989

Guppies for Tea, by Marika Cobbold, published by Black Swan, 1993

Tell me who I am again, by Linda Grant, published by Granta 1998

Younger people with dementia

Younger people with dementia: carers resource book, published by the Alzheimer's Disease Society, 1996

Index

Have you found **Alzheimer's at your fingertips** practical and useful? If so, you may be interested in other books from Class Publishing.

High blood pressure at your fingertips £11.95
Dr Julian Tudor Hart

The author uses all his 26 years of experience as a GP and blood pressure expert to answer your questions on high blood pressure.

> 'Readable and comprehensive information'
> *Dr Sylvia McLaughlan, Director General, The Stroke Association*

Diabetes at your fingertips
NEW FOURTH EDITION £14.99
Professor Peter Sonksen, Dr Charles Fox and Sister Sue Judd

461 questions on diabetes are answered clearly and accurately - the ideal reference book for everyone with diabetes.

> 'I will certainly recommend it to my patients ... I think it is brilliant.'
> *Robert Tattersall, Professor of Clinical Diabetes, Queen's Medical Centre, Nottingham*

Parkinson's at your fingertips £11.95
Dr Marie Oxtoby and Professor Adrian Williams

Full of practical help and advice for people with Parkinson's disease and their families. This book gives you the information and the confidence to tackle the challenges PD presents.

Cancer information at your fingertips
NEW SECOND EDITION £11.95
Val Speechley and Maxine Rosenfield

Recommended by the Cancer Research Campaign, this book provides straightforward, practical and positive answers to all your questions about cancer.

Heart health at your fingertips
NEW! £14.99
Dr Graham Jackson

This practical handbook, written by a leading cardiologist, answers all your questions about heart conditions.

> 'Contains the answers the doctor wishes he had given if only he'd had time.'
> *Dr Thomas Stuttaford, The Times*

Asthma at your fingertips
NEW SECOND EDITION £11.95
Dr Mark Levy, Professor Sean Hilton and Greta Barnes MBE

This book shows you how to keep your asthma - or your family's asthma - under control, making it easier to live a full, happy and healthy life.

> 'This book gives you the knowledge. Don't limit yourself.'
> *Adrian Moorhouse MBE, Olympic Gold Medallist*

PRIORITY ORDER FORM

Cut out or photocopy this form and send it (post free in the UK) to:

Class Publishing Customer Service
FREEPOST (no stamp needed)
LONDON W6 7BR

Tel: 01752 202301

Fax: 01752 202333

Please send me urgently
(tick boxes below)

**Post included
price per copy
(UK only)**

☐	**Alzheimer's at your fingertips** (ISBN: 1 872362 71 0)	£17.99
☐	**High blood pressure at your fingertips** (ISBN: 1 872362 48 6)	£14.95
☐	**Diabetes at your fingertips** (ISBN: 1 872362 79 6)	£17.99
☐	**Parkinson's at your fingertips** (ISBN: 1 872362 47 8)	£14.95
☐	**Cancer information at your fingertips** (ISBN: 1 872362 56 7)	£14.95
☐	**Heart health at your fingertips** (ISBN: 1 872362 77 X)	£17.99
☐	**Asthma at your fingertips** (ISBN: 1 872362 67 2)	£14.95
☐	**Allergies at your fingertips** (ISBN: 1 872362 52 4)	£14.95

TOTAL: _____

Easy ways to pay
Cheque: I enclose a cheque payable to Class Publishing for £ _____
Credit card: please debit my Access ☐ Visa ☐ Amex ☐ Switch ☐

Number _____   Expiry date _____

My address for delivery is

Name _____

Address _____

Town _____

Telephone number (_____

Credit card billing add _____

Town _____

Class Publishing's guara
with these books, we will
and VAT rates may be alte